50 Years of Failure

50 Years of Failure

American Healthcare Policy at a Crossroads

BROOK CHAMBERY

50 Years of Failure
American Healthcare Policy at a Crossroads

Library of Congress Control Number: 2020911503

ISBN: 978-1-7350272-1-0 (Paperback)
ISBN: 978-1-7350272-3-4 (eBook)

Printed in the United States

Edited by Alan Axelrod
Design by Carol Norton
Cover image by Shutterstock

For further information or to contact the author,
please go to www.BrookChambery.com.

"FACTS ARE STUBBORN THINGS;
AND WHATEVER MAY BE OUR WISHES,
OUR INCLINATIONS, OR THE DICTATES OF OUR
PASSIONS, THEY CANNOT ALTER
THE STATE OF FACTS AND EVIDENCE."

—JOHN ADAMS,
*Argument in Defense of the [British] Soldiers
in the Boston Massacre Trials, 1770*

CONTENTS

Introduction

The frustration with healthcare quality and cost has been ongoing for decades but has reached a tipping point. We as individuals, businesses, and taxpayers are weary of and can no longer afford price increases of three to five times the rate of inflation. We are justifiably anxious for a solution. Healthcare spending, which was 4% of GDP in 1970, is now 18% and quickly climbing to 20%.

Consumers, powerless to control anything in the healthcare realm, are floundering, struggling to keep their heads above water, especially as more of the cost has been dumped on them by way of high-deductible plans without price transparency, and whose ever-narrowing provider networks often make it impossible for subscribers to see the physicians of their choice.

Large self-insured corporations such as Walmart, Amazon, JP Morgan, and Berkshire Hathaway are trying to take matters into their own hands, moving to gain purchasing power, whether individually or through alliances. They hope to create competition for their business by doing their best to track hospital and physician data revealing quality of service and price and then attempting to contract directly with exemplary providers for needed services. On April 22, 2019, Kate Davidson cited in the *Wall Street Journal* a new report released by the trustees of Social Security and Medicare, who project that if the Medicare rate of spending doesn't change, the hospital-insurance fund will be depleted by 2026. Medicaid costs are likewise driving state and local budgets to the breaking point.[1]

Another *Wall Street Journal* article by Anne Tergesen, published the same day, discussed the anticipated 6.5% increase for Medicare Part B premiums in 2020. For those over 65, forced to join the system, forced to pay the premiums, and even forced to subsidize the premiums of others, this is especially frustrating.[2]

The pressing questions on the minds of business leaders and individuals, as taxpayers and consumers are these:

1. Why does healthcare have to cost so much?
2. Why aren't more service options available?
3. Why don't we have transparency on pricing and quality?
4. Why does healthcare appear to be so structured and inefficient?
5. Why do costs and quality vary so much?

The answers? Distressingly few exist. The assumptions are that healthcare delivery is very complex, mysteriously different than other industries, and in need of massive amounts of regulation and bureaucratic control. However, if so, why have the bureaucrats not answered the questions outlined above and solved the problems?

The solutions being proposed by politicians are generally divided into two camps. In one camp are those who assume that a single- payer system is the only solution. In the other are those who focus on a combination of "de-federalizing" aspects of the healthcare system in favor of granting states more flexibility to design their own healthcare benefit and delivery systems, as well as mandating more price transparency from providers and insurers.

The problem with the proposed solutions is that they are built on the typical assumptions and fail to take into account the structural framework of the healthcare industry, or learn from the failures in public policy implemented over the past 50 years. Thus, they are bound to fail.

A prerequisite to gaining a fresh perspective on healthcare is to recognize that the mystery and perceived complexity of this industry is actually due to the regulatory structure that has been established on the federal and state levels over the last 50 years in an attempt to control benefit usage and costs. Congress and state legislators afraid of patients and providers taking advantage of the system with inappropriate placements, service usage, and exorbitant costs, created a regulatory structure that has resulted in just that—a system out of control in usage and cost, and lacking the quality and service options consumers desire.

This book aims to expose and enlighten, debunk and demystify, and present what fifty years of history, aided by decades of Congressional reports and my experience as a provider in the industry, dictate as the obvious and most straightforward solution. It is a solution simply crying out to be embraced, and one that will lead to tremendous price reductions, quality improvements, and new service offerings. History and experience are great teachers. We desperately need to pay attention.

CHAPTER 1

The Healthcare Industry

A MAJOR AND QUICKLY GROWING SEGMENT OF OUR ECONOMY

Healthcare has become big business. The *Wall Street Journal* reported on July 31, 2018 that "The revenues of health-care companies represented nearly 16% of the total revenues of firms in the S&P 500 last year, up from about 4% in 1984."[3] On March 22, 2019, MedPac (Medicare Payment Advisory Commission), a congressional agency charged with analyzing healthcare issues and advising Congress on them,[4] reported that in 2017, the most recent data available, total national health care spending was $3.5 trillion, or 17.9 percent of our nation's GDP. Of this, $3 trillion was for "Personal healthcare spending," which is the total less spending on government health programs, administration of public or private health insurance, and medical research. It also stated that current projections are for 5.5% growth annually through 2026, at which time the total spending will be $5.7 trillion dollars, representing a staggering 19.7% of GDP.[5]

Hospital systems, which are consolidating at an unprecedented rate, as well as integrating under their control physician practices, surgery centers, urgent care centers, labs, skilled nursing services, and home healthcare services, are today among the largest employers in the United States. In 2017, according to *Visual Capitalist*, hospital systems and university systems that include hospital systems are the largest employers in 23 states.[6] This finding was consistent with two other studies by 24/7 Wall Street, reported by *Business Insider* on June 11, 2017,[7] and *USA Today* on March 30, 2019, identifying sixteen states in which the largest employers were hospital systems, and another seven in which universities that owned hospital systems were the largest employers.[8] *The Rochester Review,* a magazine published by the University of Rochester, which has a large hospital system, stated that it was not only the Rochester region's largest employer—with 27,000 employees—but it was tied for the fifth-largest employer in all of New York State. The article went on to reveal that of the top ten employers in the state, the top three are hospital systems and two other systems tied with University of Rochester for fifth place.[9] If this is the case in New York State, it is very likely that hospital systems occupy a significant number of top-ten employer positions in every state.

On June 28, 2019, the *Wall Street Journal* reported that "two major Midwestern hospital systems plan to merge ... creating another regional giant as the nation's $1 trillion hospital sector continues to consolidate." The result would be an operation totaling 76 hospitals in 26 states, along with outpatient centers, skilled nursing, and home care operations, all producing some $11 billion in revenue. These deals are "forming regional powerhouses and creating new national giants" with tremendous market power and influence over prices and quality of care. The report also cited other deals consolidating dominant systems in adjacent markets. The mergers were happening even though "growing market power and its potential effect on prices has come under greater scrutiny from health policy makers."[10]

The March 2019 MedPac report cited further evidence of the growing pace and scope of consolidation in the healthcare industry:

> Regulators and researchers have noted concerns about increased consolidations and their effect on prices. In 2015, the number of hospital mergers increased 18 percent from the prior year and 70 percent from 2010. ... The Government Accountability Office (GAO) found that, between 2007 and 2013, the number of physicians in "vertically consolidated" practices—hospital-acquired physician practices, physicians hired as salaried employees, or both—nearly doubled (Government Accountability Office 2015). In addition, the Federal Trade Commission observed that "providers increasingly pursue alternatives to traditional mergers such as affiliation arrangements, joint ventures, and partnerships, all of which could also have significant implications for competition" (Federal Trade Commission 2016). Increased consolidation has an inflationary effect on prices paid in the private sector. A recent study (Cooper et al. 2015) found that disparity in hospital prices within regions is the primary driver of variation in health care spending for the privately insured. The study shows that hospitals that face fewer competitors have substantially higher

prices, and hospital prices in monopoly markets are more than 15 percent higher than those in areas with four or more competitors. It also found that, where hospitals face only one competitor, prices are over 6 percent higher; where they face two, almost 5 percent higher.[11]

Runaway hospital system consolidation is clearly cause for concern—but not just because it is creating monopoly and/or oligopoly power throughout the American healthcare sector. The more frightening aspect of this trend is that the newly emerging health system behemoths don't even have control of their costs. The title of a 2018 *Wall Street Journal* article asked the apparently simple question, "What Does Knee Surgery Cost?" and answered, "Few Know and That's a Problem." Reporter Melanie Evans looked at Wisconsin-based Gundersen Health System, with six hospitals at the core of its network, and noted that it had no idea what it cost them to operate on a knee, one of the most common surgeries performed and one of the most straightforward when it comes to calculating cost. Yet, it took Gundersen eighteen months of work with (presumably highly paid) consultants to determine that the system's costs for this one procedure were one-fifth of their list price, which is the base for negotiations with insurance companies. Moreover, it took Gundersen over a year of internal discussions before it even launched its attempt to accurately determine knee surgery cost. Knowing the cost of producing a good or service is the alpha and omega of any business plan, and yet it was not regarded as a particularly urgent matter by Gundersen's administration. As Jess Wieser, owner of a company that is part of an alliance contracting with Gundersen, remarked, his company "tracks its own costs in minute detail ... [and] there's no reason [Gundersen] can't run a business like we do."[12]

Gundersen's mindset is not only incomprehensible and irresponsible, it is the norm throughout the nation's metastasizing healthcare systems. From all appearances, Gunderson management failed to understand perhaps the most basic principle of buying and selling anything. To price your products, you need to know the cost of your products. Moreover, by paying close attention to what is being spent, you can figure out how to be much more efficient.

The incredible thing is no one at Gundersen—neither the CEO nor the CFO—seemed in the least embarrassed about their lack of knowledge concerning the organization's operations and the prices charged to those being served in the community. On the contrary, Gundersen management was obviously comfortable having the story reported—and even proud of their leadership in finally getting a handle on this aspect of their business. Why the self-congratulatory attitude? Because the mere effort to determine costs, to gain even a modicum of control, would set Gundersen apart from its competitors, who made no such effort.

Well, the moment has not yet come for Gundersen management to break out the champagne. Knee replacement surgery is only one of 750 classification groupings for hospital inpatient stays and 800 codes for hospital outpatient services.

In the meantime, employers and consumers know only one thing for certain. Healthcare costs continue an unrelenting drive upward, with no end in sight. The growing affordability crisis will soon become universal. In 1970, healthcare accounted for 4% of GDP. It now (2018) represents 18% and, according to Med-Pac, will rise to approximately 20% of GDP in 2026, or $6 trillion dollars. Since 1960, inflation has lifted prices approximately 500%, while healthcare costs have increased around 1,600%.[13]

None of this comes as any surprise to anyone who has been paying healthcare insurance premiums and other healthcare expenses over the years. A drive around your own city will doubtless reveal the pervasiveness of ever-expanding hospitals and new business parks dedicated to physician offices, clinics, urgent care centers, surgery centers, and so on. Yet the pace of this healthcare cost inflation and industry consolidation is nevertheless both mindboggling and terrifying.

As Johns Hopkins University healthcare economist Gerard Anderson remarked in a 2018 *Wall Street Journal* report, "the marketplace is just not working." The *Journal* went on to observe that, thanks to consolidation, "hospitals can be shielded from the competition that forces other industries to wring out expenses and slash prices. … Consolidation has given hospitals greater pricing power in many markets, according to health-economics researchers."[14]

In a 2006 book, *Redefining Health Care: Creating Value-Based Competition on Results,* Professors Michael E. Porter and Elizabeth Olmsted Teisberg discussed the dysfunction they observed in the healthcare marketplace *before* the current wave of consolidations. They discerned a fundamental problem in healthcare, arguing that the structure of the care delivery system was broken because competition was broken and describing the symptoms of this condition: "Costs are high and rising despite the fierce struggle to control them. Quality problems persist. The failure of competition is evident in the large and inexplicable differences in cost and quality for the same type of care across providers and geographic areas. Competition does not reward the best providers, nor do weaker providers go out of business. Technological innovation diffuses slowly and does not drive value improvement as it should." The healthcare marketplace, they asserted, had gravitated to a zero-sum competition, in which participants compete to shift costs to one another, accumulate bargaining power, and limit services. All actors in the system share responsibility for the problem. "Taken together, these outcomes are inconceivable in a well-functioning market."[15]

"In a normal market, competition drives relentless improvements in quality and cost," Porter and Teisberg write. "Rapid innovation leads to rapid diffusion of new technologies and better ways of doing things. Excellent competitors prosper and grow, while weaker rivals are restructured or go out of business. Quality-adjusted prices fall, value improves, and the market expands to meet the needs of more consumers. This is the trajectory of all well-functioning industries – computers, mobile communications, banking and many others." Yet the authors go on to conclude that the problems in this marketplace do not flow from lack of competition, but from the wrong kind of competition, taking place at the wrong levels, and focused on the wrong problems. The way to transform healthcare and dramatically increase value, they argue, is to realign competition so that system participants are *forced* to compete on value.

The obvious problem with Porter and Teisberg's proposed solution is that they accept that the healthcare marketplace is not open but managed or controlled. Its players can be "realigned" and "forced" in various directions by the directors—namely, government officials, regulators and legislators. Their solution is not a bold reform but simply assumes more of the same interventional system manipulation that has taken place over the last fifty years—and, of course, failed miserably.

In taking this position, these professors have not even attempted the most basic marketplace analysis that would be expected of their freshmen economics students. They have failed to ask the essential questions:

- Why should the healthcare marketplace be any different from any other marketplace and thus need to be managed?

- Can management of this or any other marketplace work?

- Why shouldn't weaker rivals be forced out by competitors with stronger customer-value propositions rather than trying to train or force them to do things differently?

- What is the structural and regulatory framework of the healthcare industry?

- What barriers to entry exist?

- Who are the major payors?

- Is it the industry or the regulatory structure that creates the complexities in this market?

What has made the healthcare delivery system extremely complex and mysteriously different from other industries is simply the massive degree of regulation at the state and federal level that has been put in place over the past half-century. The majority of politicians, educators, and the public does not realize the extreme level of influence exerted by government regulatory design at both the state and federal levels.

The regulatory regime, including Medicare and Medicaid reimbursement policies and other controls have distorted the economics of the entire healthcare delivery system. Yet most people assume that because healthcare providers are private enterprises and institutions, the current system is a free, competitive marketplace. This being the case, private enterprise must be responsible for the crisis and, therefore, the crisis can be addressed only through even more regulation or a single-payer system.

This is far from reality. Although there are private entities operating in the marketplace, for all practical purposes it is government design and control that dictate how the system is structured and operates. After five decades, hundreds of legislative changes, thousands of demonstration projects, and hundreds of billions of wasted dollars, the goal of quality care in the most appropriate setting and at the best price remains as elusive today as it was in 1965.

The fact is that in 50 years under the current system we have not been allowed to experience care being delivered in any manner other than what our regulators have designed and/or allowed. Besides enduring healthcare expenditures that have greatly exceeded the rate of inflation, we don't even know what it should cost to deliver care. Government design rather than competitive innovation has resulted in a stagnant, archaic system of care delivery that leaves the consumer profoundly dissatisfied and the taxpayers bankrupt. Market disrupters have been removed, protectionism and political jockeying for market position reign, and what could be a vibrant marketplace is currently dominated by entrenched monopolistic enterprises.

Federal and state regulations control the types of providers, what services they offer, and how these services are to be delivered. Because these regulations control who can be in the business, they also control—that is, suppress—the degree of competition. They control the operating standards, quality inspections, and provider ratings. They set the rates paid for about 60% of the services rendered, and these rates influence the remaining 40%. Federal and state regulations establish and mold new directions for the industry through demo projects and financial incentives provided to meet bureaucratic expectations.

THERE COULD NOT BE A BETTER PRESCRIPTION FOR DISASTER

Taking upon itself the authority to dictate a regulatory structure for the healthcare industry in addition to creating healthcare benefits, Congress has enacted legislation that—

1. Defines the types of providers, thereby limiting innovation in service delivery
2. Mandates and enforces the standards of operation for these service providers, thereby limiting the flexibility to innovate and drive efficiency
3. Allows the states to control the number of providers and who they are, thereby limiting competition and incentives for innovation and efficiency
4. Defines and pays for a benefit not according to the medical need but by the type of setting in which service is being provided, thereby allowing inappropriate placement and services
5. Dictates the prices for the services delivered, thereby limiting the ability of market forces to make these determinations

THE MEDICARE INFLUENCE

A good deal of this book is devoted to a critical consideration of Medicare policies, which are national in scope and influence the rest of the industry. Twenty years of MedPac reports provide support for this criticism. Recall that MedPac, an agency of Congress, is tasked with analyzing access to care, quality of care, and other issues affecting Medicare. It also advises Congress on payments to health plans participating in the Medicare Advantage (MA) program and providers in Medicare's traditional fee-for-service (FFS) program. MedPac was established by the Balanced Budget Act of 1997 (42 U.S.C. 1395b-6 (2008)). The reasoning for my focus on Medicare will become increasingly evident as we continue, but the MedPac reports are also an excellent source of general information and historical perspective on the entire healthcare industry.

The March 2019 MedPac report stated that, at 25% of total spending, Medicare is the single largest purchaser of services in the healthcare system. Medicare paid for 25% of all hospital care, 30% of all prescription drugs, 40% of home health care, and 23% of skilled nursing care. The amount spent for the average Medicare recipient (16% of the population, or 57 million persons) is approximately $12,385, or 300% of that for the average working age person. Medicare spending was $705.9 billion, or 3.6 percent of gross domestic product (GDP) in 2017.[16]

A payer as massive as Medicare will have an extremely significant effect on the market, but, as the MedPac commission explains, its influence extends even further:

> Spending under Medicare's FFS [Fee for Service] payment system is used to set benchmarks for Medicare Advantage (MA) plans and for accountable care organizations (ACOs). More importantly, it is also the foundation of MA plans' payment rates to hospitals. ... In addition, the Department of Veterans Affairs began setting hospital rates equal to Medicare FFS rates in 2012 ...The rates that uninsured individuals pay are also often benchmarked to Medicare due to limits on rates charged to low-income uninsured individuals that were enacted in the Patient Protection and Affordable Care Act of 2010 (PPACA). The Medicaid program also uses Medicare rates when setting maximum supplemental "upper payment limit" Medicaid payments to hospitals (Medicaid and CHIP Payment and Access Commission 2016). Furthermore, Medicare rates can affect rates charged by commercial insurance. ... Given the growth in the use of Medicare FFS prices as a benchmark, any update to the Medicare base payment amount will affect many other payers.[17]

Because FFS has such far-reaching effects, MedPac cautions that "It is imperative that the current FFS payment systems be managed carefully ... for the unit prices established, their overall level, the relative prices of different services in a sector, and the relative prices of the same service across sectors—is of critical importance."[18]

The March 2019 MedPac report stated that, in 2017, Medicare (federal) and Medicaid (state and federal) direct outlays were 22% ($660 billion) and 18% ($521 billion) of healthcare spending, respectively. The Department of Defense (DOD), Veterans Administration (VA), and Children's Health Insurance Program (CHIP) accounted for 4% ($126B) of spending, and there was another 9% ($248B) spent by other ("third party") payers, including Indian Health Services, workers' compensation, child health, Substance Abuse and Mental Health, and other federal, state, and local programs. Since the total of all of these programs comes to 53% of all outlays, it is safe to say that another 25% of the out-of-pocket" spending (or 3% of total spending) for co-insurance and other privately paid healthcare purchases is also connected to these programs. In total, this means that government-related programs are responsible for approximately 56% of our direct healthcare spending outlays.[19]

Private insurance accounts for the remaining 40% ($1.2 trillion) of personal healthcare spending. Since 2008, commercial insurance prices, on average, have grown faster than Medicare's prices.[20] This is hardly surprising. With Medicare holding down rate increases, the hospitals try to make up the difference through price negotiations with insurance companies. Indeed, MedPac noted that a major driver of increased hospital and physician group consolidation is an effort to gain leverage over insurers when negotiating higher payment rates.[21]

There is some truth to this. The Kaiser Family Foundation stated that in 2019 seven insurers were responsible for 80% of the Medicare Advantage recipients: United Healthcare, 26%; Humana, 18%; BCBS, 15%; CVS, 10%; Kaiser, 7%; Cigna, 2%; and Wellcare, 2%.[22] It is even more significant that the top three insurers hold a 59% market share. The March 2019 MedPac report (p. 358) noted the market concentration of the top two actually went up to 55% in the non-metropolitan areas. Insurers and hospitals keep pointing the finger at each other as the party that holds the most power in contract negotiations and is thus responsible for the price increases. But the rate setters and regulators for Medicare and Medicaid? They get a free pass, and so calls for a single payer system, as in Europe and elsewhere, become increasingly strident. In the meantime, large employers, frustrated by the lack of any progress in cost control, try to force system change by taking matters into their own hands.

CHAPTER 2

1965: The Beginning

FEDERAL AND STATE GOVERNMENTS ESTABLISHED AS REGULATORS, PAYORS, AND MARKET MAKERS

In 1965, Congress passed Public Law 89-97, amending the Social Security Act and establishing the Medicare (Title XVIII) and Medicaid (Title XIX) programs. Medicare is a federal health insurance program for those age 65 and older, with hospital and post-acute services under Part A, and physician and other medical services and supplies under a supplemental Part B. Medicaid was a joint federal/state program covering healthcare for those with low incomes. The Medicaid Section of the law established "Grants to States for Medical Assistance Programs" and required that there be a State Plan for this medical assistance (Section 1902(a)(2)). The state had to contribute at least 40% toward the program cost.

Unfortunately, very little thought went into this massive legislation. Instead of broadly determining benefits and letting competition and the professionals in the marketplace determine the types of care and its cost, Congress and the executive branch went far beyond.

DEFINING PROVIDERS AND STANDARDS OF OPERATION

Under SSA Section 1861, Congress took it upon itself to define the types of providers (or institutions) and services to be recognized for inpatient reimbursement under Medicare Part A. For example, the law defined a skilled nursing facility and, for reimbursement purposes, limited its use to post-acute "extended care services"— and then only after a three-day in-patient stay at the hospital.

There are other innovative uses for these facilities than envisioned by the regulators, and if left to the expertise of industry professionals, they would have been employed to save the health system a great deal of money.

Section 1861 also instructed the Secretary of Health Care Finance Administration (HCFA) to define the conditions of participation, or standards of operation, that Medicare would require of the various providers. Section 1902(a)(22)(B) demanded the same of the states under their Medicaid authority. Section 1863 allowed the states, because of their Medicaid authority, to specify higher patient care standards than established by the secretary under Medicare. Typically, states designate that they will use the Medicare standards, but Section 1902(a)(22)(D) mandated that no matter what, their Medicaid State Plan is to define what standards they determine to use. This is very important, not only for consistency purposes, but because Section 1864 further added that the Secretary could use the state agencies to survey and determine compliance with both the federal and state standards. Section 1814(b) (22)(D) mandated that the survey methods used by the states would be dictated at the federal level.

Just as Medicare recognizes state Medicaid standards to maintain program continuity for surveying and certification, states must apply their Medicaid standards to all licensed facilities, whether or not they participate in the Medicare or Medicaid programs. With the dominant role of Medicare and Medicaid business in the market, and program certification standards enforced as state licensing standards, it is easy to see how Medicare and Medicaid regulations not only influence but control the industry. It is important to keep this in mind as we move forward.

PAYMENT STRUCTURE UNDER MEDICARE PART A

SSA Section 1814(b) dictated that the amount paid to any provider under Part A is to be "the lesser of the reasonable cost of services as determined under Section 1861(v) ... or the customary charges" for such services. State Medicaid plans (Section 1902(a)(20)(D)) also had to define the methods to be used to determine "reasonable costs." In Section 1861(v)(1)(A) Congress went on to mandate that "The reasonable cost of any services shall be the cost actually incurred, excluding therefrom any part of incurred cost found to be unnecessary in the efficient delivery of needed health services, and shall be determined in accordance with regulations establishing the method or methods to be used, and the items to be included. ... Such regulations shall take into account both direct and indirect costs of providers ... in order that ... the costs of a covered stay .... will not be borne by those not covered by the program."

In order to attempt to determine the costs actually incurred, Section 1861(v)(1)(F) and Section 1865 specified that the secretary of health and human services also develop and mandate the use of audited cost reports. Section 42 CFR 413.9(b) of the implementing regulations states, "Reasonable cost of any services must be determined in accordance with regulations establishing the method or methods to be used, and the items to be included." The same "reasonable cost" language was used for Medicaid, Section 1902(a)(20)(D) requiring that the Medicaid State Plans define the methods to be used to determine these "reasonable costs," but without reference to some of the mandated aspects in calculating the Medicare rates, thus intentionally leaving room for flexibility.

The language in Section 1861(v)(1)(A) regarding costs actually incurred and necessary, and the Section 1865 cost-reporting mandate is most unfortunate because the "reasonable cost of services" in a fully competitive marketplace would be determined by the "customary charges." In such a world, there would be no need for cost reports, audits, and rate setters. MedPac recognized this in its March 2001 report when it stated that what it should cost efficient providers to furnish services would be approximated by competitive pricing. The June 2006 MedPac report stated that a truly competitive market can identify the price that "matches the marginal cost of an efficient provider." The March 2007 MedPac report also stated that "most sectors of the U.S. economy rely on market forces to ensure the efficient allocation of resources."[23]

Section 1861(v)(1)(F) did provide a way to let market forces substitute for other methods of determining costs: "Such regulations may ... provide for using different methods in different circumstances ... [including] estimates of costs ... and may provide for the use of charges or a percentage of charges where this method reasonably reflects the costs." However, because of other licensing restrictions and barriers to entry implemented by the states, there was no competitive marketplace, and HCFA had to use cost reports, audits, and rate setting to approximate what competitive pricing *might* have accomplished. In cost report parlance, the customary charge became the private rate, or gross charge, rather than the market-clearing rate (that is, the price reached when supply is balanced with demand).

BARRIERS TO ENTRY CREATED WITH STATE LICENSING

In 1964, New York State enacted the Metcalf-McCloskey Act requiring health department officials to determine the need for new in-patient facilities and out-patient programs. A Certificate of Need (CON) would have to be issued before a facility could be built or a program started to furnish certain types of services. The logic for this law was tied to the market-distorting mandate for cost reimbursement. In other words, if regulators guaranteed provider costs, the market could easily become oversaturated with providers, which would soon lead to underutilization or excess capacity, either of which would drive up costs.

Ten years later, in 1974, following New York's lead, the federal government passed the Health Planning Resources Development Act, which required every state to establish CON programs. This meant that before any new provider could be "established" or capital projects (such as a new facility, expansion, or new programs) begun, a request had to be made to the state planning boards, who would decide whether or not to issue the required CON. The 1974 law also meant that state health departments could define which of the federally defined levels of care would be allowed in that state, as well as what additional licensing requirements would be applied as a requirement to obtain establishment approval—the CON. State bureaucrats thus became healthcare market gatekeepers, controlling the barriers to entry as well as level of competition in the marketplace and thus ultimately controlling the services available and the quality of those services.

Competition and innovation? These were, by legislative fiat, replaced with political maneuvering, protection schemes, and market stagnation. The Health Planning Resources Development Act was also a fertile breeding ground for corruption. In belated recognition of this, in 1987, the federal government dropped the health-planning requirement. Nevertheless, as of 2019, thirty-five states, Puerto Rico, the US Virgin Islands, and the District of Columbia still retain CON laws. Some of the other states cling to remnants of the federal law they hold dear.[24]

The thing is, once regulatory controls become entrenched, it is incredibly hard to get rid of them—even, as in the case of the CON laws, the federal government eventually recognized the error of its ways. The bureaucrats who run the state programs join the providers (who are eager to protect their comfortable market positions) and fight hard for the status quo. In his September 14, 2011, Civitas Institute article, "Certificate Of Need: Did It Actually Control Healthcare

Costs?" Neil Inman noted that even "a sustained push for repeal by the Department of Justice during the Bush years" could not dislodge the program.[25]

The June 2006 MedPac report stated, "Truly competitive markets can identify [a price that matches the marginal cost of an efficient provider] but health care markets are imperfect because of asymmetric information, moral hazard, adverse selection, and limited supplier competition among other factors. Medicare generally sets the prices it will pay for services administratively." However, it is the CON programs and other licensing controls that have been limiting the competition and preventing "the use of charges or a percentage of charges where this method [could] reasonably [reflect] the costs" as allowed by Section 1861(v)(1)(F), thereby creating the need for rate setting. The March 2007 MedPac report stated, "We rely on competition among producers and service providers to keep prices in check while they make the goods and services that society wants. Within most sectors of the economy, this interaction of demand and supply leads to prices that act as signals of how much society values a good or service relative to other uses and thus determines how resources are allocated."[26] We have lost the ability to allow these market forces to take root in the healthcare marketplace.

There is simply no excuse for assuming the healthcare marketplace is functionally any different from any other sector of the economy. In its March 2007 report, MedPac cites the arguments that are typically put forward[27]:

1. "Patients often do not know what specific health services they need or the relative benefits and costs of treatment options. They rely on physicians and other providers in a principal-agent relationship, who help make decisions on their behalf. While professional codes of conduct should guide providers toward furnishing appropriate care, providers do not necessarily have the same motivations and preferences as their patients."

I believe most patients would—or certainly should—take great exception to this typical bureaucratic and regulatory mindset. People want to exercise control over their own healthcare decisions, including their choice of providers, on whom they rely for information.

2. "Unlike sectors of the economy that produce standard products, health care providers must individually evaluate the symptoms and conditions

of patients to tailor plans of care, and they must do so in the face of uncertainty about the best course of action. As a result, it can be difficult to evaluate the quality (including appropriateness) and efficiency of a specific provider's care and build consensus among providers around standards of care."

Many segments of the economy involve individualized or customized solutions for each client—and function just fine. The need for individual customization is hardly unique to healthcare and therefore does not stand up as an argument for arbitrary regulation of who can be a healthcare provider. The proof? This rationale has consistently worked very poorly indeed.

3. "Most health care services are financed through insurance," which is beneficial, but "also shields patients from seeing the full cost of their care. This can lead individuals on the margin to use more and higher priced services than they would otherwise—particularly since they rely on providers to help decide what care they need."

This statement assumes that insurers are not interested in the best outcomes for their enrollees, including those "on the margin," or that they and the providers cannot become involved with—or are simply unconcerned about—determining the best and most efficient course of treatment. These assumptions are both unwarranted and ridiculous.

MedPac's concluding argument is bound up with misguided policies and regulatory structures that have been in place since the late 1960s, as we have discussed. MedPac asserts that, in the healthcare industry, "lack of competition among certain types of suppliers can lead to relatively high prices for their products or services and little pressure to improve efficiency over time." The failure to realize the irony of this statement is astonishing. It is the regulators who are chiefly responsible for the lack of competition in many healthcare sectors, and distorting markets by administratively determining prices. As MedPac goes on to state, "Mispricing of services can lead to misallocation of investment resources, which can have large effects on the organizational structure and cost of health care delivery over time." In a normal free market, high prices would inevitably lead to more competition and lower prices.

Outpatient Services (Medicare Part B)

Part A is an entitlement program, funded by mandatory Social Security and Medicare tax revenues, which support the Medicare Trust Fund. Part B, in contrast, was established as a "Supplemental Medical Insurance" program funded by premiums paid by the beneficiary, with the remainder coming from general tax revenues. Part B covers Medical and Health Services, defined under Section 1861(s) to include outpatient physician visits, supplies, orthotics, drugs, occupational therapy, physical therapy, surgery, and so on. The reimbursement pendulum swung in completely the opposite direction for Medicare Part B services, the focus changing from reasonable *costs* to reasonable *charges*. The problem is that the law fails to define "reasonable charges" in Section 1861—or anywhere else, for that matter. Thus, in the implementing regulation at 42 CFR 405.502, HCFA states that the "law allows for flexibility." It then goes on to list many criteria for making such determinations, including customary charges, prevailing charges, or, if the quality of product or services does not vary "significantly," the lowest charge at which services, supplies, and equipment are available in the area. It also states (at (b)) that the charges recognized cannot be higher than would be paid for comparable services provided under the same circumstances. Nevertheless, under (h), there are acceptable corridors for variations in provider charges.

The Unbelievable Lack of Analysis in Establishing Medicare and Medicaid Legislation

We can debate the wisdom of regulation in general, regulation in particular areas, or particular regulations. What cannot be debated or otherwise disputed, however, is the promulgation of regulations without an underlying basis in careful analysis. Regulations have the force of law and powerfully affect markets as well as the state of healthcare availability and quality. Such powerful legislation and rule making cannot be based on assumptions, guesses, mere policy and politics, or whims. And yet, the legislation governing Medicare and Medicaid rests on a staggering paucity of analysis.

Medicare
Before enacting Medicare, Congress had debated a variety of proposals for government health insurance programs for decades. Throughout, the legislators

29

encountered heavy resistance from hospitals, physicians, and insurers alike, all of whom strenuously opposed what they regarded as an intrusion into the industry by "socialized medicine." Their response was to advocate for the expansion of the role of private insurance, with private subsidies for lower-income patients.

Lyndon Johnson, vice president under John F. Kennedy, assumed the presidency after JFK's assassination on November 22, 1963, and ran for election in his own right in 1964, achieving a landslide victory against conservative Republican Barry M. Goldwater. LBJ enjoyed a Democratic majority in Congress, a bulging Social Security Trust Fund, and, as the faithful steward of what he portrayed as the social vision of the martyred Kennedy, the popular momentum to finally get the government health insurance job done. The issue of government health insurance took on a more serious legislative tone. Wilbur Mills, the Republican chairman of the House Ways and Means Committee, who had previously been skeptical of all this additional government spending allied with the Democratic president as the major forces behind what became Medicare.

To advance their cause, the bipartisan pair acceded to the demands of the major players in the healthcare industry. Hospitals wanted to ensure that their costs, including those for providing charity care, were covered. Physicians, who resisted any form of government control, were looking for continued reimbursement based on *customary* charges. Insurance carriers, who desired to maintain their business, wanted to serve as fiscal intermediaries for Medicare. As politicians, they also desired wide acceptance of the program by insurance carriers. For they quite correctly worried about the ability of the Social Security Administration to adequately administer the program.

In a 1995 article, "What Medicare's Architects Had in Mind," Robert Ball, who had been a commissioner of Social Security under Presidents Kennedy, Johnson, and Nixon, wrote: "We did not propose a program to reform the health care delivery system. ... We did not intend to disrupt the status quo. Had we advocated anything else, it never would have passed. Thus, the bill we wrote followed the principles of reimbursement that hospitals all over the country had worked out with the Blue Cross system." Likewise, "Part B was explicitly based on a private insurance plan, an Aetna plan for federal workers under the Federal Employees Health Benefits Program (FEHBP)." This is confirmed by the March 2007 MedPac report, which states that "Policymakers designed Medicare's benefit structure and its payment methods to look like private insurance that was available at the time."[28]

He went on to say it was intended that "Hospitals would be allowed to nominate an intermediary to do the actual work of bill payment and to be the contact point with the hospitals. Government would be unobtrusive. The carrot was that many hospital bills that had previously gone unpaid because the elderly had no money would now be paid."[29] By and large, the government's posture at the beginning was one of paying full costs and not intervening very much in how hospitals, at least the better ones, conducted their business. In fact, the first section of Title XVIII of the Social Security Act, which provided for health insurance for the elderly, was a "Prohibition Against Any Federal Interference ... or the exercise of supervision or control over the practice of medicine ... or over any institution, agency or person providing health services."

According to Bob Rosenblatt, President Johnson knew speed was of the essence if he was to enact this comprehensive legislation, and, indeed, passage came in just seven months after the bills were introduced in the House and Senate.[30] Wilbur Cohen, whom President Kennedy had appointed as Assistant Secretary of Health, Education and Welfare for Legislation, helped to design and pilot the legislation through Congress. In his "Reflections on the enactment of Medicare and Medicaid,"[31] Mr. Cohen stated that ideological and political issues were so dominating that they precluded consideration of such issues as reimbursement alternatives and efficiency options. Things moved so quickly that Mills only allowed him one day to prepare a draft of the voluntary insurance plan to cover physician services. This is confirmed by Robert Ball, who wrote ... Part B had been added to the administration's hospital insurance plan at the last moment by Wilbur Mills. ... We had only one weekend in which to try to adapt the Aetna plan to a government-run plan."[32] Cohen recalled:

> It was a strange and unique way in which to make a major policy decision. There was no policy clearance with others in the Department or in the Budget Bureau or White House. ... I was the intermediary for a major expansion of our proposal without any intervening review of the details of the proposal as developed by the staff. In this case, the Federal Government was moving into a major area of medical care with practically no review of alternatives, options, trad-offs, or costs. ... For me, at the moment, the big question was not on the method of reimbursement to physicians but rather on the "voluntary" nature of Part B. ... Moreover, no one on the Committee raised any questions about the radically new principal of using Federal general revenues – equal to 50

percent of the cost of the plan. We felt that such a subsidy would be necessary to make a voluntary plan accepted by low-income retire people. As I recall it, no major question arose in the House, Senate, or Administration on this unexpected addition of Part B.

Mr. Cohen continued, "Successful implementation of Medicare required the cooperation of hospitals, physicians, nurses, carriers, intermediaries, and other providers. The primary objective was to get off to a good start. ... One feature that I built into the legislation was making the effective date July 1, 1966. ... We needed every day of the approximately 11 months we had to prepare for putting the law into effect."

Concerning reimbursement policy, Mr. Cohen's statements get even more astounding: "The hospital part of Medicare had been in one or another stage of staff discussion since 1942 ... many different versions of such legislation had resulted in pinpointing administrative and policy questions." Yet—

> The principle of "Reasonable Cost" for in-patient hospital services embodied in section 1814(b) and 1861(v) of the Social Security Act was never seriously debated or opposed during the period 1961-65, as far as I can recollect. ... No one criticized it during the legislative process as a "cost-plus" principle. No one thought of it as a basis for inflationary price or cost rises. It was accepted not only because no other alternative was proposed, but because conventional wisdom at the time accepted reasonable cost as a reasonable principle.

The provision in the legislation that "the Secretary shall consider, among other things, the principles generally applied by national organizations" helped in getting Congress and providers to accept the focus on reasonable costs.

As Wilbur J. Cohen and Robert M Ball put it in "Social Security Amendments of 1965: Summary and Legislative History":

> The Secretary of Health, Education, and Welfare is required, to the extent possible, to contract with carriers to carry out the major administrative functions of the medical insurance plan, such as determining rates of payments, holding and disbursing funds for benefit payments, and determining compliance and assisting in utilization review. No contract can be entered into by the Secretary unless he finds that the carrier will perform its obligations efficiently and effectively and will meet requirements, such as those relating to financial responsibility and legal authority and other matters as the Secretary finds pertinent.
>
> The contract must provide that the carrier take necessary action to see that, where payments are made on a cost basis, the cost is reasonable. Where

payments are on a charge basis the carrier must see that such charge will be reasonable and not higher than the charge applicable, for a comparable service and under comparable circumstances, to the carrier's other policyholders and subscribers. In determining reasonable charges, the carriers will consider the customary charges for similar services generally made by the physician or other person or organization furnishing the covered services and also the prevailing charges in the locality for similar services. Payment by carrier for physicians' services will be made on the basis of a receipted bill or an assignment under which the reasonable charge will be the full charge for the service.[33]

This analysis is confirmed in the March 2007 MedPac report, which states, "policymakers designed Medicare's benefit structure and its payment methods to look like private insurance that was available at the time. An important provision within Medicare's statute precludes the program from 'exercising any supervision or control over the practice of medicine.'" However, "at the time, the health insurance industry was in its infancy."[34]

Medicaid

The programs implemented in 1965 included another element: Medicaid. Momentous, it was nevertheless billed as a rather insignificant federal expansion of a program already in place to help states pay the medical bills of the poor. As Wilbur Cohen put it:

> Many people, since 1965, have called Medicaid the "sleeper" in the legislation. Most people did not pay attention to that part of the bill (...under the heading of "Improvement and Extension of Kerr-Mills Program"). Title XIX was not a secret, but neither the press nor the health policy community paid any attention to it because of the dazzling bewilderment of the adoption of Part B. ... The full awakening to the scope of the Medicaid legislation did not come until much later. The health policy community in 1965 was a small band of brothers and sisters concerned about the controversial elements in Medicare and unaware of the possibilities inherent in Medicaid. But the idea of Medicaid developed in my mind as early as 1942. I waited for the right time when someone would ask me to develop it into a law. The year 1965 was that time.

Earlier. Cohen stated that "All during the years 1960-65, I took the position that both Medicare-type and Medicaid-type programs were necessary and desirable and were not in conflict with each other. Mr. Mills readily accepted this view."[35]

In a 2011 Harvard University undergraduate thesis, *Selling Medicare, Forgetting Medicaid,* Stephen George Anastos wrote:

Once the omnibus measure left Ways and Means, with help from labor, the bill moved through the Rules Committee – usually a hang-up for controversial legislation – in just a day and a half. On the House floor, all the publicity surrounding Medicare monopolized debate … Republicans accurately complained that the debate was really a "farce" … The opposition was correct in its assessment that no one really understood what the bill contained, but even Republicans did not understand just how little everyone knew. Their opposition was aimed at the more controversial Medicare, allowing Medicaid to enter the package unchecked.[36]

Anastos went on to note that President Johnson "afforded just a single sentence to Medicaid" in his remarks at the signing of the omnibus Social Security Amendments. A bill decades in the making, Medicare received all the attention, and it took a few months for the states and the media to wake up to the gold mine that was the Medicaid legislation. On February 7, 1966, *The New York Times* admitted that Medicare had gotten all the attention, but officials were saying that Title XIX "is the opening shot of a revolution—the beginning of a new style for the nation's medical services."[37]

As New York jumped in to grab an expected 300% increase in federal dollars, a group of upstate legislators urged the Department of Health, Education, and Welfare to bar the program New York proposed. "Rarely has social legislation of the scope and cost of the state's new medical care program been enacted amid such confusion or set in motion with so little sense of direction. It is evident now that many legislators voted for the program with virtually no understanding of its significance."[38]

New York's planned program drew an avalanche of criticism from across the country. The *Chicago Tribune* criticized New York for setting in motion "the most elaborate program of state medicare in the nation despite increasing criticism that the legislation is going too far in the direction of socialized medicine."[39] The state's program was set to spend more than Congress had allocated for all of Title XIX, and the three most expensive state plans already were projected to be 2.5 times the anticipated federal Medicaid budget in the first year. This led to urgent discussions behind closed doors in the U.S. House Ways and Means Committee, but it was too late to reverse course. The expansion was only just beginning.

Regarding the principles of paying for medical services under Medicaid, Wilbur Cohen explained, "With the acceptance of "reasonable cost" in Title XVIII, I arranged for the inclusion of 'reasonable cost' in section 1902(a)(13)(B) of Title

XIX." Yet he did so while omitting the constraints in section 1861(v) under Title XVIII "on the assumption that this would give the Secretary and the State somewhat greater flexibility in a State-by-State administration of Title XIX." Section 1902(a)(13)(B) provided for payment of reasonable cost "as determined by the Secretary" of Health, Education, and Welfare instead of actually specifying the principles or methods to be followed. Mr. Cohen noted that the explanation given to members of the Ways and Means Committee was that "payment of comparable reasonable costs in Title XIX would upgrade medical services to the needy and assist in carrying out the 'amount, duration, or scope' of equality of treatment requirements in section 1902(a)(10)." It was an explanation Chairman Mills accepted "enthusiastically."

A HUGE BUREAUCRACY IS SET IN MOTION

Federal Medicare and state Medicaid cost reporting methods and forms had to be developed, the elements of reasonable cost had to be defined, and appeal mechanisms established. Rate setters, auditors, appeals officers, and attorneys had to be hired. The details regarding types of providers, levels of care, and operating and quality of care standards to be followed in providing care had to be defined. Survey (quality of care inspection) procedures had to be developed for enforcing the standards and certifying providers. Surveyors had to be hired and trained. Survey appeal mechanisms had to be established. Regulations and operations manuals had to be developed at both the federal and state levels for all of this.

Since the federal government retained final control over the state Medicaid programs, it also had to establish the regulations, operations manuals, and legal mechanisms governing contracts with the states, controlling various services provided by the states and other contractors (such as for surveying activities), and mechanisms of reporting the costs of state operations, auditing those reports, and reimbursement of the costs. The same level of overhead had to be established at the state level to control dealings with the federal government.

Once such a massive bureaucracy is designed and in place, it takes commensurately massive legislative efforts to change it. In fact, it has never been changed. In the September 2018 issue of Hillsdale College's periodical *Imprimis*, John Steele Gordon wrote that "more than 90 percent of the medicine being practiced today did not exist in 1950."[40] Yet, the structure of our healthcare delivery system has been stuck in time, existing today much as it was designed by law and regulation in 1965.

In a March 1, 1999 AEI (American Enterprise Institute) article, Robert Helms cites Ball's 1995 article (cited above) to the effect that after-the-fact reimbursement for hospital costs was a clearly flawed policy. He then continues: "As health economist Ted Frech points out, this attempt to adopt the practices of the private market as they existed in 1965 was already out of date even as Medicare was being implemented. The private market was beginning to move away from cost-based reimbursement, while the Medicare legislation locked the government program into a historical straitjacket."[41] Although, as we will see, the government moved away from cost reimbursement, the industry is still plagued by government-established pricing and regulatory controls. The regulatory straitjacket fashioned in the 1960s by a government with little vision and less knowledge still controls the healthcare industry today.

CHAPTER 3

1972: The Adjustments Begin

ROLLING INTO RATE SETTING

I n his 2006 article, "The Origins, Development and Passage of Medicare's Revolutionary Prospective Payment System,"[42] Rick Mayes recalled a conversation with William Hsiao, who had begun his career in 1969 by examining hospitals for the Social Security Administration (SSA) and, later, in the 1980s, spearheaded the development of Medicare's fee schedule for physicians. In that conversation with Mayes, which took place years after Medicare was implemented, Hsiao recalled the hospital industry's opposition to being required to adopt standard accounting procedures. He told Mayes that he wondered why hospitals were getting paid cost, plus two percent. In fact, he could not figure out how hospitals even calculated their costs. Unable to get the answers from hospital administrators, Hsiao was left to "discover" for himself that there "was no uniform accounting system or anything close to it" and that the "government paid the hospitals based on what Blue Cross was paying."

What the hospitals had worked out with Blue Cross was retroactive cost reimbursement. Hospitals had an even sweeter deal with the commercial insurance companies, which based their reimbursement on hospital charges—ordinarily, higher than costs. Mr. Mayes stated that although the SSA pushed, "we could not make the hospitals adopt uniform accounting systems." Thus, in the early years, there was no way to even estimate reasonable costs, as mandated in the Medicare legislation. Congress had gotten the legislation passed with the backing of the hospital industry by informally stating that it would pay the "usual, customary and reasonable" fees, a method used by Blue Cross plans, and then adding 2%. The result? From 1966 to 1973, healthcare spending rose by an average of 11.9% a year.

DEVELOPMENT OF COST REPORTS

By 1972, the government had developed and mandated a standardized accounting and reporting system for Medicare, and the states began doing the same for Medicaid. At the end of the fiscal year, all providers were required to submit audited financial statements and cost reports on mandated forms. These reports were used to determine the allowable costs of running the facility, including breakdowns by department, patient days, tests administered, therapies delivered, and so on to derive a cost-per-unit of service.

The data was the basis for any retroactive settlement necessary to adjust for the difference between costs and the interim payments received throughout the year. It would also be used to establish provisional rates for the next fiscal year. Since a profit factor was not allowed, a return on equity, or interest on invested capital, was included as part of the costs reimbursed. Thus, if all the costs were categorized as allowable, the facility administration could plan on at least getting reimbursed for cost plus a return on the equity invested. Since a business also needs to more than cover costs to survive in the long term, the system was dependent on subsidy by higher rates from whatever other private or insurance business the provider could arrange. The ability to do that, of course, depended on the quality of the service produced by the provider. But under this system, unless the provider was extremely incompetent, it was virtually guaranteed that revenues would cover costs plus a return on investment. This environment invited both fraudsters and those who had no knowledge of healthcare. But it led to a huge boom in the industry.

FROM REASONABLE COST TO REASONABLE-COST RELATED

In an attempt to further limit cost increases, Congress passed the all-encompassing 1972 Social Security Amendments, which, among other things, authorized the secretary of what was then called the Department of Health, Education, and Welfare (HEW) to undertake experiments and demonstration projects with the goal of limiting payments. The 1972 legislation thus authorized much more flexibility in developing formulas for determining reasonable costs for inpatient hospital services, establishing limits on what was considered a "reasonable" cost, setting prospective reimbursement rates, developing payment options for durable medical equipment, and requiring a three-day hospital inpatient stay before allowing reimbursement for skilled nursing services.

For nursing homes, the legislation even allowed the states to vary from "reasonable cost" to "reasonable cost-related" reimbursement, using cost finding techniques and methods approved by the secretary. These provisions eventually led to numerous and wide variances in Medicaid reimbursement formulas at the state level, which were intended to limit the costs a given state recognized as "cost-related." For instance, besides establishing cost limits, New York abandoned standard accounting principles where it was advantageous, such as substituting mortgage principal payments for depreciation expense. New Jersey, in concert with consultants from Yale University, developed the first Prospective Payment Systems (PPS), which would later become the model adopted for national use.

The comprehensive 1972 legislation went beyond payment mechanisms and further defined and regulated providers. It established a single definition of a skilled nursing facility (SNF), mandated certification requirements and operational standards for such facilities, and specifically identified the services SNFs could and could not provide. The legislation also outlined inspection requirements for hospitals and SNFs and established provisions for the monitoring of Medicaid and Medicare fraud.

In 1973, Congress passed the Health Maintenance Organization (HMO) Act and authorized the loans and grants necessary to get these organizations established. HMOs were envisioned as another mechanism for controlling costs, and beneficiaries were encouraged to sign up accordingly. This was followed by the Stabilization Act of 1975, the intent of which was specifically to limit the rate of rise in hospital fees. Yet, as Mayes noted, despite all these efforts, hospital "costs" went up 345% between 1966 and 1976, almost four times the CPI increase, which was 89% during this same period.

When the Health Care Financing Administration (HCFA), which is now Centers for Medicare and Medicaid Services (CMS), was established in 1977 within the HEW (which is now HHS, Department of Health and Human Services) to take over supervision of Medicare and Medicaid, costs were already double what they had been in 1975. By 1980, costs were *three* times what they had been in 1970. A crisis was brewing. An article published in *The Balance* on November 14, 2018, pointed out that, from 1974 to 1982, costs had continued to rise by an average of 14.1% a year, and the program was projected to quickly crowd out discretionary spending in the federal budget.[43]

As Mayes recounts, the Reagan Republicans were anxious to get control of hospitals, doctors, and insurers but doubted the effectiveness of any private market solution, including forging a deal between the politicians and the industry to voluntarily contain costs. It was at this point that New Jersey's experimental prospective reimbursement model was proposed as a model for a national system. Without any solid data to substantiate the success of this New Jersey waiver program, without any modern computers to crunch the numbers, and with only a preliminary analysis of the program by Yale and Rutgers, the concept was sold to an eager Congress.

PROSPECTIVE REIMBURSEMENT FOR HOSPITALS

In 1982, Congress passed Public Law 97-248, the Tax Equity and Fiscal Responsibility Act (TEFRA), and the Prospective Payment System (PPS) became law for hospital reimbursement under Medicare. The March 2000 MedPac report stated that "increasingly, policymakers recognized the limitations of the [retrospective] cost-based reimbursement ... and of administered pricing in general. To varying degrees, policymakers sought to develop prospective payment systems for providers currently subject to cost reimbursement." According to Mayes, the hospital industry was having a hard time dealing with the cost limitations applied over the past few years and felt that they could get by under PPS. As MedPac noted, "In general, expected PPS benefits included a more aggregate unit of payment that would remove the incentive to add services to a particular episode (of care) and a prospectively determined rate. That meant providers could keep the rewards if they cut their costs. [The] PPS system also provided policymakers with a tool to control spending directly, through base payments and updates."[44]

Thus, PPS became the solution to a political problem, and Congress, again without debate or any understanding, made it law. Mayes quoted Republican senator Bob Dole's healthcare aide, Sheila Burke: "We all knew only too well the impact of any change in Medicare could lead to seismic changes in the industry, because Medicare was such a big purchaser. We were all enormously sensitive to that, and also enormously sensitive to not really knowing how to defend or describe what appeared to be real differences between hospitals, their costs and their mix of cases. We knew far less than one would have hoped about what would occur after making these changes."[45]

The 1982 legislation added Section 1886, which stated that the secretary was not to recognize any costs as reasonable that exceeded a certain percentage above the average for all hospitals in the same group. Groupings had to consider the mix of patients and services, type of hospital, and geographic area. Diagnoses were used to form patient-mix characteristics and were then weighted according to the expected or estimated relative resources that consultants determined would be necessary for their care. The consultant studies were to rely on quizzing nursing or other medical staff to get their thoughts on the use of resources for various case-mix categories, and the cost calculations were to be done by applying the weighted scale to costs taken from a certain base year and on a budget-neutral basis. The resulting cost figures would then be projected for a certain rate year using desired trend factors as opposed to actual cost changes taking place in the industry or economy.

PPS was felt to be a great way to control cost increases. Why? Because the base year, cost limitations, and trend factors could all be manipulated by the bureaucrats according to budget constraints. As for the hospitals, however, not only did they survive under PPS, they became more adept at working around it—even as the PPS reimbursement system was further refined to accomplish its cost-controlling goals.

By the late 1980s, hospitals had experimented with patient rehabilitation and found that, contrary to traditional thinking, the service could be rendered in their skilled nursing facilities rather than a hospital setting. This created a huge opportunity. Hospitals could discharge patients much sooner by transferring them to their own skilled nursing facilities for rehabilitation in a *post-acute* setting. Since the PPS rate was based on the total expected stay, which Medicare had envisioned as including *in-hospital* rehabilitation, the hospital corporations could now get paid twice. While maintaining the hospital-level PPS rate, they could transfer the patient to the rehab center and begin collecting at the daily rehabilitation rate. The result? The number of hospital-based skilled nursing homes (SNFs) almost doubled between 1991 and 1997, and hospital profit margins grew significantly.

The increase in hospital margins continued as independent skilled nursing facilities also joined the shift to rehabilitation services. In fact, the March 2000

MedPac report noted that hospital profit margins were six times higher in 1997 than they had been in 1991—because of these transfers to post-acute settings for rehab.[46]

The March 2001 MedPac report stated: "Policymakers expected the use of post-acute care to grow when the prospective payment system (PPS) for inpatient hospital services was implemented in 1983 ... however, use of post-acute care grew much more rapidly than expected; between 1988 and 1994, Medicare spending for post-acute services increased at an average annual rate of 34 percent."[47] Spending on nursing homes during this period also went up—by more than 400%. SNF spending increased explosively, from $2.5 billion in 1990 to $11.3 billion in 1996. The number of people receiving care in SNFs doubled, and the per-day cost tripled, largely as a result of the increased use of such ancillary services as physical and occupational therapy. Even though a profit factor is not an element found in the SNF Medicare rate structure, we can assume that the rates that were being established appeared sufficiently inviting to draw many into offering rehabilitation services. If policymakers believed SNFs were not only capable of delivering rehab services and doing so more cost effectively than in a hospital setting, we can only wonder why they had not so empowered the SNFs earlier.

Even as skilled nursing homes were reducing hospital usage, advances in medicine were reducing the length of hospital stays, and patients were making use of their Medicare homecare benefits. The March 2000 MedPac reported: "In 1997, Congress faced a Medicare program with an annual growth rate of more than 8 percent; some sectors, such as home health, had annual growth rates of more than 30 percent. ... The increase in home health and SNF spending also raised concerns about whether cost-based reimbursement was creating incentives for overutilization and, in turn, excessive spending. Home health spending nearly quintupled in six years, going from $3.5 billion (3.5 percent of Medicare spending) in 1990 to $16.9 billion (8.8 percent) in 1996. The numbers of home health agencies, beneficiaries being served, and visits per beneficiary all increased, as did evidence of management problems, fraud and abuse, and the provision of unnecessary services (Grob 1997)."[48]

The growth in post-acute care services led Congress to direct HCFA to replace cost-based payment methods with prospective rates for post-acute services.[49]

PROSPECTIVE PAYMENT FOR ALL PROVIDERS
(1997 – PRESENT)

MedPac reported in March 2000 that HCFA's assessment was that, overall, the PPS implemented for hospitals in 1983 led to reduced spending for hospital services and increased efforts by hospitals to control costs. Thus, "benefits were expected from extending PPS payment systems to other services, such as home health, SNF, hospital outpatient, and hospitals not already covered by the current PPS system, including rehabilitation and long-term care hospitals." In 1992, HCFA implemented a physician fee schedule, which set payments for services in advance and was thought to have succeeded in limiting aggregate spending growth.[50]

The Balanced Budget Act of 1997 (BBA) and the Balanced Budget Refinement Act of 1999 (BBRA) launched "profound changes in Medicare's payment policies," mandating prospective reimbursement throughout the industry. It was at this point that "HCFA responded to these mandates, adopting new payment systems for services furnished by skilled nursing facilities (SNFs), hospital outpatient departments (OPDs), and home health agencies. In addition, the agency modified its payment systems for hospital inpatient care and physician services while developing new PPSs for inpatient rehabilitation facilities, long-term hospitals, psychiatric facilities, and ambulatory surgical centers."[51]

With the 1997 legislation, Congress ended the Medicare "reasonable cost" era by redefining what was meant by *reasonable cost*. The elements of cost considered reasonable for reimbursement did not change, but just as we described earlier regarding the original hospital PPS system, limits would now be applied in three major ways.

- First, limits were applied by choosing the "base year" from which the costs would be taken and then applying agency-determined inflation factors instead of recognizing the *actual* cost increases a provider or region might have experienced.

- Second, for most of industry segments, HCFA had to define categories of patients or services, estimate the relative differences among them in costs (labor, supplies, overhead, and so on) of delivering the service for each group, derive the average cost of service in a defined region for a

43

particular base year, and multiply this by the relative value scale to set a rate for each category patient or service.

- Third, HCFA would determine what inflation factor would be applied to base year costs to derive a current year rate.

The providers, still required to submit annual cost reports, effectively supplied HCFA with the data necessary to shop for the best base year. HCFA could— and did—retain the use of certain base years, simply updating the annual trend factors, if doing so was deemed favorable. Tweaking the rates in this manner was, in theory, an effective budgeting and cost-control tool. The states quickly followed suit in establishing their Medicaid rates. To give an example, as of 2020, SNF rates are still set using allowable costs from 1995 cost reports, the same base year used to establish the 1998 rates, which was when the PPS first became effective for SNFs. Thus, for over twenty years, CMS has avoided acknowledging any structural changes and actual cost increases that might be reflected in using a more current base year. During this period, CMS has gone from 44 to 66 diagnosis related groupings, and as late as October of 2019, continues to tweak the system even further.[52]

The March 2000 MedPac report noted that the BBA and related policy changes were expected to slow the growth in payments, saving an estimated $112 billion between 1998 and 2002. These savings, combined with a shift in the financing of many home health services from Part A to the Part B trust fund, extended the projected depletion date of the Hospital Insurance Trust Fund by about six years—through early 2007.[53]

The MedPac Commission summed up the achievements of the Balanced Budget Act of 1997 (BBA) this way:

The legislation achieved reductions in provider payments ... across provider groups. One recurring policy change reduced the annual update adjustment for providers paid under existing prospective payment methods. This policy was enacted for inpatient hospitals, physicians, and managed care plans. Another type of policy change created new PPSs for providers previously paid under cost-based reimbursement, which allowed Congress to adjust the new payment components under these systems to produce savings. ... A third mechanism reduced formulaic payment adjustments; capital, indirect medical education, bad debt, and disproportionate share adjustments were all reduced to hospitals. ... Reductions in provider payments accounted for about $99 billion of the estimated Medicare savings. Another $13 billion was saved through an increase in beneficiary premiums, which resulted from an increase in the percent of Part B costs paid by premiums and from the transfer of many home health services from Part A to Part B.

The commission added a caveat, however: "Despite its unprecedented magnitude, the BBA did not fix the long-term financing needs of the program. Instead, it created the savings necessary to allow Congress more time to consider appropriate longer-term solutions for Medicare that would address the fundamental mismatch between spending projections and expected revenue growth."[54]

Yet: "Within two years—before many BBA provisions had been put in place, and before the Congress was ready to address long-term Medicare reform—provider groups persuaded the Congress to revisit many BBA provisions and issues. These groups were concerned that many provisions had unintended consequences and that access to some Medicare services might be compromised. The result was the BBRA." The commission went on to explain that the BBRA of 1999 was projected to increase spending by about $16 billion over five years by making adjustments in the payment formulas across provider categories, but this was just a small fraction of the $1.3 trillion expected to be spent by Medicare over the 2000-2004 time period.[55]

The BBRA was followed by the Benefits Improvement and Protection Act of 2000 (BIPA), which addressed inadequacies in the wage index calculations made in deriving the PPS rates. To get an idea of the level of complexity with which HCFA had to deal under PPS, the BBA mandated that the wage index (discussed earlier) be calculated separately for each of the 374 individual regions around the country. When even this level of granularity was subsequently judged inadequate, the BIPA directed the agency to further refine its input by collecting and weighting data by occupation. Provider rates would then be further adjusted by category of provider and the typical percentage of staff employed in the various occupations.

Simply incredible.

CHAPTER 4

The Rate Setting Nightmare

EXPECTING THE IMPOSSIBLE

As the March 2002 MedPac report acknowledged and as the last chapter discussed, the Balanced Budget Act of 1997 (BBA), the Balanced Budget Refinement Act of 1999 (BBRA), and the Medicare, Medicaid, and SCHIP Benefits Improvement and Protection Act of 2000 (BIPA) "fundamentally changed the way Medicare pays for many products and services."[56] These laws required the Health Care Financing Administration (HCFA) to modify the hospital prospective payment system (PPS) and develop and adopt new prospective payment systems for services furnished by skilled nursing facilities (SNFs), hospital outpatient departments, home health agencies, rehabilitation facilities, long-term care hospitals, and psychiatric facilities. The laws also required CMS to change the method by which prospective capitation payments were made to health care insurers under the M+C (Medicare+Choice) program. The BBA also mandated a competitive bidding demonstration (CBP) for durable medical equipment (DMEPOS).

HCFA already had a huge responsibility. As the March 2002 MedPac noted, "Medicare's 40 million beneficiaries use thousands of different health care products and services furnished by over 1 million providers in hundreds of markets nationwide."[57] Rates had to be established for everything: physician services, acute care, emergency and outpatient services, post-acute services, hospice care, labs, drugs, durable medical equipment, etc. The March 2014 report furnished a snapshot of the mindboggling scope of the infrastructure that HCFA was, and is dealing with, most of which is subject to regional wage index, inflation, and a myriad of other adjustments:

- 749 patient diagnosis related groupings (DRGs) for hospital inpatient care, with various complex exceptions for outlier cases
- 800 ambulatory payment classification groupings (APCs) for hospital outpatient care (The March 2018 MedPac report counted approximately 700 outpatient codes.[58])
- 66 DRGs for skilled nursing
- 153 DRGs for home health
- 44 DRGs for Inpatient Rehab Facility (each further adjusted by functional motor skills, cognitive ability, age, and length of stay)
- 749 DRGs for long term care hospitals (The LTC-DRGs are the same DRGs used under the hospital inpatient prospective payment system [IPPS], but they have been weighted to reflect the resources required to treat the type of medically complex patients characteristic of LTCH stays.)
- 3,700 procedures in the Healthcare Common Procedure Coding System (HCPCS) for ambulatory surgery centers
- 7,000 services in the physician fee schedule (PFS), for physicians and other clinicians who perform procedures in various hospital, outpatient, or physician office settings. If procedures are predominantly performed in a physician's office, the physician is paid the same as if done in the ambulatory surgery center.
- The services of the other medical personnel and medical supplies involved with the above procedures, which are included in a bundled payment system linked to the hospital outpatient and surgery center payment systems. Payment varies by whether services were performed in a physician's office, urgent care center, emergency department, and whether on or off the hospital campus.

Setting and maintaining accurate payment rates across many health care settings in hundreds of local markets, the March 2001 MedPac report noted, is a tall order for several reasons:

Providers' costs are difficult to determine. We have little or no information about costs for most types of health care professionals—physicians or independent therapists, for example. The available measures for facility providers, such as hospitals and nursing facilities, are based on accounting costs, which may differ from true economic (resource) costs.

Most health care providers and plans produce multiple products, many operate across two or more settings—hospital inpatient and outpatient services, for instance—and virtually all serve many patients or beneficiaries covered by other payers, making it difficult to isolate costs associated with specific services furnished to Medicare beneficiaries.

Adjusting payment rates to reflect the effects of local market conditions—differences in input prices, for example—requires knowledge of providers' production processes and cost components, and accurate data (that are often not readily available) for related market factors.

Medical science and technology and local market conditions are continually evolving; thus, payment rates must be frequently updated to maintain consistency with changes in efficient providers' costs.[59]

"It is difficult to distinguish the effects of payment policies from those associated with changes in technology, beneficiaries' preferences, or diffusion of new care standards. ... Correctly interpreting these trends is challenging ... Available information is often incomplete—we usually lack accurate measures of providers' overall product mix, for example. We lack the ability to control for changes in care quality. Finally, the information we have is based on accounting costs, which may differ substantially from true economic costs because allocations of fixed and overhead costs are arbitrary and because unit costs measure average rather than marginal costs. ... All of these measures present formidable challenges of interpretation. Consequently, none of them provides conclusive evidence about the appropriateness of Medicare's base payment amounts in any setting."[60]

"The lack of adequate monitoring tools and data is a major problem, especially in a period of rapid change. ... the tools and data available in the short run may suffer from so many limitations that policymakers should carefully consider whether prospective payment is appropriate. ... prospective payment is not always better. If the products Medicare is buying cannot be well defined and monitored, payment rates are likely to be seriously inaccurate."[61]

The March 2001 MedPac went on to observe that, in addition to all the problems cited above:

> HCFA cannot do everything at once. ... Developing and implementing new payment systems is a difficult and time-consuming task in the best of circumstances; adopting five or six new systems nearly simultaneously is unprecedented. Given the volume of work [with all the new mandates], HCFA lacked the staff resources and time to fully prepare new payment systems and make the necessary changes in its administrative systems. Some objectives that could have been addressed in less hectic conditions were sacrificed, including prior development of monitoring systems to track changes in provider behavior that might adversely affect beneficiaries.[62]

As one example, the Committee commented on the post-acute care prospective payment systems that had been established: "Because these new systems focus on the settings in which care is provided rather than the care itself, they raise concerns about whether Medicare's payment policies are appropriate."[63]

The March 2001 report commented: "Designing, developing and implementing four different PPSs for the interrelated parts of post-acute care is a major challenge because effective systems would pay correctly not only within settings but also across settings." The BIPA (Benefits Improvement and Protection Act of 2000) added to these problems by mandating the development of patient assessment instruments with comparable common data elements on the premise that there was potential overlap across these post-acute services, a premise which, MedPac stated, is not supported by empirical evidence.[64] Twenty years later, this task has yet to be accomplished.[65]

MEDPAC POSES POLICY FRAMEWORK
QUESTIONS YET TO BE ANSWERED TODAY

The March 2001 MedPac report stated, "Our policy framework suggests important questions that should be asked about any payment system." The first question? "Is the product or service that Medicare is buying well defined and does HCFA have sufficient ability to monitor product attributes so that fixed-price contracting is desirable?" Another important question: "[I]s the current level of the payment rates consistent with the costs efficient providers would incur in furnishing covered services to beneficiaries."[66]

The March 2002 MedPac Report observed: "To set and maintain accurate payment rates for many products and services—even in a single setting—is a difficult task. At a minimum, policy makers need certain tools," including "complete knowledge of the products and services Medicare is buying, the production processes used by providers, the inputs that contribute to efficient service, and beneficiary characteristics and market circumstances that may affect costs." The report went on to caution "that judging payment adequacy involves substantial uncertainty; for many settings, the available data are not current, indicators are often ambiguous, and the health care industry continues to change rapidly. ... we have no compelling evidence that payments [in 2002] are too high or too low."[67]

The March 2001 MedPac report warned: "Limitations in knowledge, tools, or available data ... may impair HCFA's ability to define the products it is buying or set payment rates consistent with efficient providers' costs, leaving substantial uncertainty for both sides," and, a year later, the March 2002 report admitted that "Medicare's payment policies and methods are often seen as extremely complex, a perception strengthened by the myriad policy changes enacted in recent legislation. Even without these changes, however, Medicare's size and scope—buying a full range of health care products and services from many different types of providers in hundreds of markets nationwide—would make its payment methods complicated."[68]

"Medicare continues to struggle to find appropriate methods to pay for new technologies (in outpatient settings) that ensure beneficiaries' access to new services but that do not place undue financial burdens on taxpayers and beneficiaries. Very few market data are available to set payment rates for new technologies, particularly for innovative products with patent protections," the 2002 report grimly observed.[69]

MedPac stated in March 2001 that, given the "limitations" it enumerated, "it is difficult" (a year later, the March 2002 report would escalate this to "nearly impossible") "to identify efficient providers and practically impossible to measure their short-run marginal costs. Further," the 2001 report continued:

> If all payers set their payment rates equal to efficient providers' short-run marginal costs, some providers would face insolvency because they would be unable to cover their fixed costs. As a result, policymakers usually set the initial payment rates in Medicare's prospective payment systems based on providers' historical average or median costs per unit and then rely on the incentives for efficiency inherent in predetermined payment rates to encourage providers to control their costs.[70]

In short, MedPac effectively concluded that the answer to the questions it had put forth in 2001 is no: the agency did not and could not know what products and services it was buying and what it should cost the efficient provider to furnish them. The March 2001 report further noted—drily—"In principle, these conditions would be met if Medicare's payment systems established payment rates approximating the competitive prices that would prevail in the long run in local health care markets."[71]

It is simply incredible that Congress, with over two decades of failed policy, did not stop, change directions, and give competitive pricing a chance. It was absolutely ridiculous and futile to continue to expect a regulatory body to establish and maintain reasonable rates for such a panoply of products and services, distributed across the nation and under widely varying market conditions.

BY 2007, THE SITUATION HAD NOT IMPROVED

After many years under PPS, the March 2007 MedPac report announced the obvious: "Medicare and other purchasers of health care in our nation face enormous challenges for the future." First, there is "wide variation in the quality and use of services within our health care system." Medicare "spends widely different amounts for beneficiaries across geographic regions," and "there are also wide geographic disparities in the quality of care beneficiaries receive" without any "relationship between quality of care and spending." Second, "spending has been growing much faster than the economy" for all purchasers of health services. In fact, the report warned, if adequate steps are not taken, Medicare's need for financing "will place an increasing liability on beneficiaries ... crowd out resources for other federal priorities, and potentially affect the federal budget deficit, the level of federal debt, and economic growth. ... Strategies ... [must] include using payment policy to obtain greater value."[72]

The commission recognized that the case-mix categories used for prospective reimbursement "often do not accurately track differences in the costs of care" and that the system has "changed the pattern of service use within" different healthcare settings. It also recognized that the regulators do not have "adequate data to evaluate whether beneficiaries are being treated in the setting that provides the most value to them or the program." Nor can regulators determine whether better provider financial performance "results from higher efficiency or from differences in the mix of patients chosen for treatment."[73]

The commission went on to admit, yet again, that keeping administered prices accurate is very challenging, for as Ginsburg and Grossman found in 2005, "Over time, inaccuracies and lags in the timeliness of data that CMS uses to set payment rates can accumulate into significant mispricing and unintended overpayment for certain services at the expense of others."[74]

MedPac went on to observe that economists, researchers, and other knowledgeable observers wonder why health care providers do not emulate managers in other industries by making use of current IT and systems engineering methods to increase efficiency and quality of service. The commission's conclusion was that start-up costs and lack of return on investment, as well as the "difficulty of implementing unfamiliar systems," hinder such implementation.[75] However, this simply smacks of an overprotected industry, insulated from the competition that exists in other industries. Without competition, there is none of the incentive that compels virtually all other businesses to computerize and promote continuous quality improvement. The bottom line on regulation is that, across forty years, regulators had learned almost nothing about the industry they were tasked with controlling, and they failed to understand why things were not functioning as efficiently as they should or, more to the point, as efficiently as they do in other industries.

THE COMMISSION'S CONTINUING REFUSAL
TO RECOGNIZE THE OBVIOUS

As of its March 2007 report, the MedPac Commission's remedy was to perpetuate the status quo, to double down, to keep control in the hands of government regulators, and to use "payment policy to obtain better value."

"Policymakers can better use Medicare's payment systems to create incentives for higher quality and greater efficiency. The list of approaches that policy makers might use is long: Building in incentives for providers to furnish high-quality care and to coordinate care, and setting payments for larger bundles of clinical services are just a few examples." The report went on: "CMS, along with accreditation and provider organizations has begun to play a critical role in building the infrastructure to move to pay for performance. The agency identified and developed quality measures, collected standard data on quality, and published information on the performance of some providers. It also designed demonstration programs to test various aspects of paying for improved quality and efficiency."[76]

The commission stated that its goal was to tighten standards, make payment rates more accurate, develop consensus about appropriate uses for new medical technologies, and provide incentives for quality and efficiency using payment systems that it establishes. In sum, it was not about to let the market take the lead in addressing the problems. The commission allocated just two sentences to the possibility that free-market competition could be an option—and then only within the context of addressing the implementation of a competitive bidding trial for certain durable medical equipment in various parts of the country.[77]

IN A SIGNAL OF WHAT WAS COMING ...

Suddenly, the MedPac Commission appeared to blame *the market*—or some absence of control over it—for the *government's* lack of achievement over the years:

> To ensure that a pay-for-performance strategy is successful for Medicare, CMS must continue to work with other payers and stakeholders so that the measures the agency uses are accepted widely. ... Medicare can and should take the lead in initiating certain changes. In many situations, Medicare must often work in collaboration with other payers to make lasting changes.[78]

Acknowledging that "Medicare heavily influences many aspects of health care," the commission was now more determined than ever to play its heavy hand. Never mind that the Medicare statute forbids the program from "exercising any supervision or control over the practice of medicine," the commission was in effect signaling its intention to build a case for Congressional approval to allow it virtually complete control over the health care industry in the name of achieving efficient pricing.[79]

Yet, after sending this signal, the very same MedPac report revealed just how lost the regulators were in their efforts to control the system. The commission judged the adequacy of hospital payments by whether more facilities had opened than closed, by growth in the volume of services offered, and by the level of construction spending. The report claimed that hospital payment indicators were positive even though Medicare margins in 2005 had been calculated as negative: -3.3%. The very same kind of faulty analysis was used to evaluate payment adequacy for physicians. Even though the commission continued to note "several problems" with the current pricing system, especially the inadequacy of Medicare rates for primary care services and the disparities that can be created in services offered, it considered only current beneficiary access and the ratio of Medicare to private rates as a proxy before claiming that the indicators of payment adequacy were stable.[80]

Concerning post-acute care, the 2007 report commented:

> While the PPSs (prospective payment systems) have changed the pattern of service use within each setting, we do not have adequate data to evaluate whether beneficiaries are being treated in the setting that provides the most value to them and the program. Three barriers undermine the program's ability to know if it is purchasing high-quality care in the least costly PAC (post-acute care) setting consistent with the care needs of the beneficiary: (1) Case-mix measures often do not accurately track differences in the costs of care, (2) There is no common instrument for patient assessment across PAC settings, which makes it difficult to compare costs, quality of care, and patient outcomes, and (3) There is a lack of evidence-based standards of care. Similar barriers limit our ability to assess differences in financial performance within each post-acute setting. We do not know if better financial performance results from higher efficiency or from differences in the mix of patients chosen for treatment.[81]

The truth was that neither the regulators nor the commission knew how consumers value services and quality, the price at which providers could deliver the services, and what alternative delivery systems might develop if providers and consumers were freely interacting in a competitive, market-clearing industry.

THE SEEDS ARE PLANTED FOR FURTHER INDUSTRY CONTROL

The June 2008 MedPac report was optimistically titled "Reforming the Delivery System." It began by stating: "Recent studies show that the U.S. health care system is not buying enough of the recommended care, is buying too much unnecessary care, and is paying prices that are very high, resulting in a system that costs significantly more per capita than in any other country." To this it added that marketplace barriers create "fundamental problems" for both public and private payers, and that, "As a major payer, the Medicare program shares in these problems." In thus painting Medicare as a victim, the agency refused even to consider whether it and other regulatory provisions had any part in creating marketplace barriers. The March 2009 report stated that these "challenges facing Medicare require addressing the incentives and organization of the health care system at a fundamental level."[82]

The commission went on, in that 2008 document, to continue building its case for the fundamental-level changes it intended to recommend. The authors recited the hoary bureaucratic dogma that the more capacity supplied, the more services would be consumed, and that rewarding providers individually rather that collectively for an episode of care leads to "fragmentation in the delivery system" and lack of teamwork and accountability. As the commission saw it, financial incentives had to be realigned to create change in organizational behavior. It was a position eerily in lockstep with the view of the professors discussed in Chapter 1.[83]

The 2008 document pushed ahead with neither reservation nor qualification, repeating the old and erroneous premise that "A fee-for-service (FFS) payment system … fuels economic incentives for providers to increase the volume of medical services they furnish."[84] As discussed in Chapter 1, a more careful analysis would have shown that the FFS payment system failed to work precisely because of the current structure of the healthcare system, with its regulatory constraints, barriers to entry, Medicare/Medicaid price-setting, and lack of proper incentives.

Nevertheless, the report soldiered on, citing a "need for greater accountability and care coordination" and then boldly, based on no experience whatsoever, set forth the concept alluded to in prior years, that a "reformed" and "ideal" Medicare payment system would pay for care "that spans across provider types and time." This, therefore, "would hold providers accountable for the quality of care and the resources used to provide it, … even if the resources were provided by others."[85]

Continuing its slide down this forty-year-old pipe dream, unjustifiably confident in its bureaucratic solution, the report declared that the "ideal" system would be one in which policymakers would be able to set accurate rates and pass on to providers the data needed to help them furnish better care. The authors never considered the alternative: that, given proper market freedom, competition would lead to cooperation between providers where justified, resulting in increased efficiency and quality, more innovative care delivery, and lower prices.

The commission went on to note "profound gaps in information on provider costs, quality measures, and appropriate clinical practices," which posed major barriers to healthcare reform. These it blamed on "market failures in the current health care system," including the lack of competition, rather than failures by policymakers who control the marketplace and establish the rates. The authors of the report used this perceived market failure as an excuse for bureaucratic failure, namely that "payment rates (set by Medicare) for individual products and services may not be accurate." The report nevertheless admitted that past recommendations as to encouraging use of comparative effectiveness of medical services, linking quality and payment, and attaining accurate payment haven't worked. True to bureaucratic form, the commission blithely moved on to its assertion that fixing the *Medicare system* required reorganizing the entire *health care system* at a fundamental level. It proposed a "new" direction that would supposedly pay for care across provider types and time, holding providers accountable for quality and resources consumed, and creating integrated systems that reward value. Specifically, the commission laid out three "delivery system reform concepts": medical home, bundled payment, and accountable care organizations (ACOs). It was convinced that these innovations—none of which were, in fact, new—would promote "joint responsibility" and "could" lead to better quality.[86]

THE MEDICAL HOME

The medical home was meant to be a clinical setting to serve as the central resource for a patient's primary care and the coordination of ongoing care. The principle provider, the primary care physician, would be responsible for the health of the beneficiary over time, was expected to improve quality of service, and would receive a monthly fee. MedPac recommended a pilot project that would employ primary care physicians to coordinate or manage care for those with chronic conditions to test "the hypothesis" that this model of care could be more effective and "enhance the role of the primary care practice." The commission considered this concept "a promising intervention for beneficiaries with multiple chronic conditions" even though, in the past, "Medicare [had] invested considerable effort and money in programs to engage external third-party disease management companies and private health plans" and produced only "equivocal" results."[87]

Among the initiatives productive of "equivocal" results was the Medicare, Medicaid, & CHIP Benefits Improvement and Protection Act of 2000. It established the first pay-for- performance initiative, offering incentives to entice the creation of physician group practices (PGPs) to see whether they could improve on processes to achieve better outcomes and lower costs. The participants were ten very large group practices, or integrated delivery systems. The pilot project ran from 2005 to 2009, after having devoted 2001 to 2004 to gathering the necessary base year comparison data. According to CMS, the project resulted only in "evidence of a small reduction in the rate of assigned beneficiary expenditure growth in the demonstration's five years, relative to contemporaneous comparison group expenditure growth." The dollar figure was "$171 per assigned beneficiary per person year." Even this modest reduction, CMS admitted, might have been due to other pre-demonstration market expenditure trends that continued into the demonstration timeframe. They may have made results appear better than they actually were. Furthermore, all CMS could claim in quality improvement were "notable differences over time for individual PGPs."[88]

The fact that these were large group practices, which had been granted the freedom to choose what business practices to target, should again have raised a caution flag before any headlong move into a wider application. Nevertheless, the commission recommended testing this "clinician-centered care coordination on a large-scale basis" to "hasten the testing process" and determine results more quickly, even though it "recognize[d] that there are legitimate concerns about moving quickly to a large-scale pilot." The commission rationalized that current cost and quality problems meant that the "status quo" was itself "extremely risky."[89]

In moving heedlessly forward, the commission ignored a higher priority and more fundamental problem with the Medicare physician payment structure and the destabilizing effects that it could have on the market. Since March 2002, MedPac had been recommending "improvements to the process for reviewing the relative value of physician services" and in March 2006 recognized that the commission must still "continue to examine [physician pay for performance] initiatives in future work" because it appeared that primary care services were "being undervalued." Although the 2007 MedPac report concluded that "access to physicians is generally good," the 2008 report observed that, over the past year, beneficiaries "were more likely to report difficulty finding" a primary care physician. If this was indeed the case, it would seem only logical to prioritize solving this potentially very serious problem before moving to a new demo project experimenting with how these physicians are utilized.[90]

BUNDLED PAYMENTS

The bundled payments concept went like this: "Medicare would pay a single provider entity (composed of a hospital and its affiliated physicians) an amount intended to cover the costs of providing the full range of care needed over the hospitalization episode," and the providers involved would be required to "develop new ways to allocate this payment among themselves." Without any persuasive rationale, this was blithely promoted as a more "flexible" arrangement, which, "ideally," would give "providers a greater incentive to work together." For this reason, the commission declared that it held "great potential"— even though (the report noted) "history suggests that it may be difficult to structure incentives to encourage physician-hospital clinical integration that controls resource use." The commission therefore recommended an "incremental approach" to the reform because of the "complexity associated with" it.[91]

Much the same caveat could be applied to the integration of post-acute providers into the bundled payment. This step, also promoted, had absolutely no precedent and proved to be fraught with legal and financial problems. MedPac declared itself to be "under no illusion that the path of policy change outlined here will be easy," adding that "with such significant change in incentives for an industry as complex as health care comes the possibility of unintended consequences and design challenges." Yet, rushing in where angels feared to tread, the commission again rationalized the approach by observing that the "status quo is unacceptable" while also nevertheless admitting that the "current payment system is fueling many of the troublesome aspects of our health care system."[92]

A May 2010 American Hospital Association (AHA) Research Synthesis Report stated: "the idea of bundled payment has been gaining traction for many years" and "with promising results." But it acknowledged that only "a handful of models have been implemented," all of which are "narrow in scope," and these focused on "specific conditions with defined timeframes, defined services, isolated episodes, and based in specific care settings, such as integrated delivery systems and academic medical centers." Given these conditions, the report concluded that the "design and results" of the bundled payment programs "are not necessarily generalizable on a wide scale," adding that "there is currently limited data on how to design and administer bundled payments." The AHA report concluded that, "while the concept of bundled payment is appealing, implementation is complex." Then came the most salient point: "It is telling that so few bundled payment programs have been established over the past 20 years."[93]

The AHA report dived deeper. "Past demonstration and pilot projects," it observed, "have centered on bundling payments for services provided by hospital and physicians. ... As bundled payment is proposed for other medical, chronic, or long-term conditions, it will necessitate that other providers be included ... including but not limited to: primary care physicians, home health, nursing home, long-term acute care, rehabilitation, and other providers across the full continuum of care. ... Establishing linkages between different types of providers and providers from different organizations will be a challenge." In addition, "in order to successfully undertake the function of care coordination, the entity would have to effectively work with hospitals, physicians, and other care providers to hold them accountable for high quality and efficient care delivery. Currently, few organizations have the infrastructure and influence to undertake this function."[94]

The AHA report alluded to bundled payment programs going as far back as 1987, including the Ingham Medical Center's partnership with a physician for knee and shoulder surgery; a Medicare Heart Bypass Center Demonstration (1991-1996); Medicare's Cataract Surgery Alternate Payment Demonstration (1993-1996), in which only 3.7% of eligible providers even indicated a willingness to participate (according to Abt Associates 1997); and Geisinger Health System's ProvenCare for non-emergency coronary artery bypass graft. None of these programs went beyond partnerships between the physician and the hospital, and each applied to highly specific procedures.

The premise behind the bundled care concept under the current FFS system is that providers often act independently of one another and have no formalized means for collaborating, much less for sharing financial risk. MedPac stated in 2008 that, since ("ideally") payment systems should motivate cooperation, bundling payments "may be the best way" to achieve collaboration. However, the AHA's report found that "Cost reduction and quality improvement ... results from several factors such as provider adherence to guidelines, elimination of waste and utilization reduction, and physician-hospital alignment." Moreover, it concluded that it was "still unclear which of these factors has the greatest impact on cost reduction and quality improvement."[95]

Based on my personal experience in the SNF rehabilitation business, successfully coordinating post-acute care with independent hospital and home care organizations, it is abundantly clear to me that MedPac was and remains wrong about the need for bundled payments. In my experience, even though providers were paid separately, each of them nevertheless effectively coordinated patient care across the network as needed. Working together, we formed and maintained a highly efficient, cost-effective process, which was of significant benefit to everyone: Medicare, the insurance companies, and the patients. This care coordination, which included the development of joint protocols for complex cases (such as post-cardiac surgery care), was formed quickly and adjusted as necessary. My experience proved to me that highly successful cooperation does not require common ownership or bundled payments. It simply calls for proper incentives and competition.

Thus, Glenn Hackbarth, who served as MedPac chairman from 2001 to April 2015, was wrong to state in his covering letter to the March 2010 MedPac report: "Payment reform will often require reorganizing the delivery of care, a complex and time-consuming activity in its own right," that could take years into the future to accomplish.[96] If the barriers to entry into the marketplace were eliminated and providers allowed to properly compete, what Mr. Hackbarth envisions as taking years would be worked out in months.

ACCOUNTABLE CARE ORGANIZATIONS

The goal of the ACO is to "promote accountability for quality and resource use over an extended period of time for a population of patients. Under the ACO, physicians and other providers are encouraged to work together and improve care coordination" and to "control growth in the volume of services provided." The ACO concept was also envisioned as a model that "could complement medical homes, which in some cases may be too small to support full accountability, and [bundled payments,] which creates no incentive to control the volume of initial admissions."[97]

The ACO concept is very similar to the organizations promoted by The HMO Act of 1973, which was responsible for feeding (and funding) a frenzy of activity to set up managed care organizations. Hospitals responded by either setting themselves up as HMOs, to both finance and deliver services, or to integrate with other providers to increase bargaining power with insurance companies. Thanks to a lack of adequate management expertise and the tremendous risks involved with such ventures, the hospitals soon disbanded their attempts at financing healthcare, but, over the years, they have continually attempted to build their provider networks and integrated services to increase their negotiating clout with insurers and large employers. State governments and private industry groups have also mounted numerous demo projects as experiments in managed care for chronic conditions and specific populations.

In 2008, MedPac identified as a "key lesson from the 1990s" the fact that providers' responses to financial incentives will result in structural changes in the health care delivery system," and added that the physician hospital organizations (PHOs) of the 1990s produced no measurable effect on either quality or efficiency. Yet, MedPac continues to hold out the hope that, this time, the dynamics might be different and, with the "appropriate incentive," it may be possible that these organizations will focus on quality and efficiency and not be formed simply to gain market power over Medicare and others. The basis for this hope is that, with such current regulatory constraints as anti-kickback rules, hospitals are now employing physicians, and the "literature suggests" that the salary model may be "more likely" to meet with "modest improvements" in unifying management and influencing physician behavior. But, MedPac warns, there are still "clear cautionary signs from the 1990s," and achieving agreements on how to divide revenues or manage care will be a "challenging and contentious process."[98]

WEAK FOUNDATIONS

What stands out in the 2008 report is the boldness with which new concepts are promoted—concepts that could result in tremendous structural changes to the market—not on the basis of meticulous study but on mere "literature reviews," hunches, and the willful decision to ignore past outcomes, pilot programs that produced inconclusive or manifestly unsatisfactory results.

Another example of such folly is the commission's conclusion—and that of CMS and the GAO—that the current PPS payment system for SNFs fails to reflect facility costs for nontherapy ancillary services and, in fact, provides incentives to supply more therapy than is needed. This situation had prompted the commission in 2007 to hire the Urban Institute to "develop an alternative PPS" but then to express concern that the system developed "would have a financial incentive to furnish less therapy than may be clinically appropriate." In addition,

MedPac stated in June 2008: "Relative to the current PPS, we estimate that the revised design would increase aggregate payments to hospital-based SNFs and nonprofit SNFs, and would reduce payments to freestanding SNFs and for-profit SNFs."[99]

Yet again, the bureaucrats acknowledged that "Accurate nursing cost information is key to measuring cost differences in care needs across patients" but admitted that, "in developing these payment system changes, our work was hampered by inadequate information on patient diagnoses, the services furnished during the SNF stay, and nursing costs." Hence, the flaw in the 2007-2008 PPS study. The June 2008 report went on the reveal: "CMS gathers staff times on individual patients that are used to establish the nursing component relative weights. These studies are expensive to administer and therefore are undertaken only periodically with a sample of facilities. Since the PPS was implemented in 1998, CMS has collected these data only once and the study's results are not expected until later" in 2008. In addition, MedPac cited the need for more accurate information about patient diagnoses and comorbidities (the simultaneous presence of two chronic diseases or conditions in a patient), and the desire for more information about daily changes in services and costs over the course of a patient's stay. Despite these recognized data insufficiencies, the commission simply floated yet another idea for a "pay-for-performance" program, this one involving the monitoring of change in assessment from admission to discharge.[100]

It is time for Congress to end what has become an endless series of adjustments to the system without proper knowledge of the market. These continue to have disastrous consequences for both the market and the consumer.

Rationalization for Bureaucratic Control of the Whole Marketplace Comes into Focus

As we have seen, by March 2009, the commission stated that "the challenges facing Medicare require addressing the incentives and organization of the health care system at a fundamental level." Perhaps the final layer of the commission's thinking on this matter is reflected in the covering letter to the March 2010 MedPac report, in which Chairman Glenn Hackbarth stated that "reorganization of how care is delivered may be necessary for payment reform to work." In other words, the inability to get control of Medicare costs *in the past* justified taking control of the whole healthcare system *in the future*.[101]

This thinking had already been reflected in the drafts of the Affordable Care Act (ACA), which Congress passed the very month the MedPac report appeared. Not only must we again emphasize that the original Medicare statute precludes the program from "exercising any supervision or control over the practice of medicine," but the ACA's concept of government control of an industry is in opposition to our whole free enterprise system.

Due to the lack of any successful track record or industry knowledge within CMS, Mr. Hackbarth acknowledged that radical reorganization will not be a "ready panacea" and "new payment models have to be tested and refined."[102] In sum, the bureaucrats were not giving in, and the endless adjustments to the system would continue—only now with even bigger stakes laid on the table: massive structural transformations of the whole health care marketplace.

CHAPTER 5

The ACA Enactment

CONSOLIDATING BUREAUCRATIC CONTROL

I am indebted to John Cannan's "A Legislative History of the Affordable Care Act: How Legislative Procedure Shapes Legislative History" for much of the material in this chapter, which describes the type of cram-down-the-throat legislative process and limited legislative debate used to enact the Affordable Care Act as was earlier used to enact the Medicare and Medicaid legislation and the Prospective Payment System updates.[103]

Mr. Cannan wrote:

> ... the debate over health care was contentious from the legislation's inception, and enacting it required a variety of ad hoc procedures. ... That the ACA does not fit into the traditional model of legislating is evident from the fact that it was not one single health care bill that became law, but two—the initial health care legislation, the Patient Protection and Affordable Care Act (PPACA), and the Health Care and Education Reconciliation Act of 2010 (HCERA), passed almost immediately after the PPACA to amend that legislation. ... Both chambers began working on health care in the early months of 2009, with the House taking the lead. ... Speaker of the House Nancy Pelosi released a "discussion draft" proposal for health care reform on June 19, 2009. ... On July 14 the committee leaders introduced House bill 3200—America's Affordable Health Choices Act of 2009. ... Committee leadership now usually drafts a bill outside the markup process, behind closed doors, and this is what happened with House bill 3200. ... Thus, the intensive committee discussion of the form legislation should take no longer occurs. ... Three versions of House bill 3200 were finally reported to the floor on October 14, 2009, ... The delay was apparently due to an agreement with the Blue Dogs not to rush a chamber vote, as well as a general unwillingness not to proceed until the Senate had produced its own

bill. ... The history of House bill 3200 came to an end as its three versions languished on the House Union Calendar ... and a new bill was introduced to carry the House's health care provisions to the next legislative step. Though procedurally the bill was at a standstill, House leaders were working behind the scenes throughout the late summer and fall to "blend" the separate versions together.... On October 29, 2009, the House's health care bill switched tracks with the introduction of House bill 3962, the Affordable Health Care for America Act. The new bill was the culmination of negotiation among different factions of House Democrats [and] resembled its predecessor, House bill 3200 in many ways. ... [However, it] was not referred to committee for any substantive review. It was not even listed on the House Union Calendar, which would make the bill eligible for consideration by the House. Yet it was called up on the House floor on November 7, 2009, less than two weeks after it had been introduced. The means to accomplish this feat were drawn from the many tools House leaders have to set agendas and advance legislation considered to be of greatest importance. ... The House Rules Committee moved the health care bill to the floor via House resolution 903. ... It waived all points of order, set the time of debate for several hours, and called for a vote once debate was concluded. ... The substantive components of House resolution 903 incorporated myriad changes to House bill 3962, which had been crafted during the ongoing negotiations between House Democratic leaders and various factions of the Democratic party. ... House resolution 903 passed the House in the early afternoon of November 7, 2009, after an hour of debate. House bill 3962 was passed at 11:15 that same evening, after four hours of scheduled debate. It was received in the Senate three days later.

Under traditional legislative history, the Senate should have sent the House bill to committee for consideration and markup, after which it would have been reported to the floor for a vote. If the Senate approved the House bill as passed, it would then go on to the President for his signature. If not, the bill would be returned to the House for its concurrence or to request a conference. None of these events took place. As it would turn out, the Senate would take the lead in shaping the form the ACA was to take. ... House bill 3962 was never referred to a Senate committee ... If a senator objects to further proceedings on the bill after two readings, the legislation bypasses committee review and goes on the Senate Calendar of Business, where it can be called up for floor consideration.

As the *Washington Post*'s Glenn Kessler wrote on June 22, 2017:

The key work on creating the Senate version of the ACA was done in secret. ... Working secretly in his office [with White House representatives and other Senators], ... Senate Majority Leader Harry Reid (D-Nev) merged the two committee bills and unveiled his own version of a health-care bill ... that was scored by the Congressional Budget Office. In a bit of legislative maneuvering, Reid offered his text as an amendment to a completely different House bill ... This bill (3590) had been sitting on the Senate Calendar of Business, avoiding the need for Reid to obtain unanimous consent to bring it up. This bill was also already obsolete – the issue had been taken care of in another bill – and so it was an ideal vehicle to start debate on the Senate floor. Reid inserted the text into the shell of the old bill. ... Once the deals were in hand, Reid on Dec. 19 revealed a manager's amendment revising the proposed bill, which was also scored by the CBO. He filed three successive cloture motions to end debate ... He also filed three other amendments that had the effect of "filling the amendment tree" – cutting off opportunities for the Republicans to alter the text. ... Reid pushed forward with a vote ... Republicans cried foul. "I do not remember, in my 15 years in Congress both in the House and in the Senate, any major piece of legislation such as this being debated and ultimately brought to a final vote within such a short period of time," declared Saxby Chambliss, at the time a senator from Georgia. ... Over three successive days the Senate took a series of votes ... Washington was snowbound, and delaying tactics by Republicans meant votes took place as late as 1 a.m. ... Final passage came with a 7 a.m. vote of Christmas Eve morning. ... All told ... there were about five days of consideration for the final bill in the Senate. ... The floor debate was mostly for show, an exercise designed to allow the closed-door negotiations that shaped the final bill to take place. Once the deal was struck, Reid pushed the final draft forward with as much speed as possible. ...

The late David Broder, the fair-minded Washington Post columnist, was scathing in his criticism of the spectacle in a column headlined "Health Reform's Stench of Victory." Reid, he wrote, "reduced the negotiations to his own level of transactional morality. Incapable of summoning his colleagues to statesmanship, he made the deals look as crass and parochial as many of them were—encasing a historic achievement in a wrapping of payoff and patronage."[104]

Cannan stated that one of the final housekeeping acts was to rename the bill the Patient Protection and Affordable Care Act. He also stated that "Conventional legislative history would suggest that the next step would be a conference committee. ... It does not appear to have been seriously considered as an option. ... [for this] would require overcoming potential filibusters, giving Republicans more opportunities to stall, if not thwart, the legislation. Democrats were eager to pass a bill as soon as possible ... So, instead, Democratic congressional leaders and White House officials met in what one article described as a 'substitute for a Congressional conference committee' to draft a proposal that could pass both houses. The negotiations were held behind closed doors, which raised transparency concerns and meant that this important stage would leave no record aside from what was reported in the press."[105]

In the meantime, as Cannan explains, Democrats lost their filibuster-proof majority in the Senate and faced Democratic resistance in the House as to some of the Senate provisions. Instead of giving up on this legislation, which they considered to be more politically expensive, they "went ahead with a complicated but often used parliamentary practice that would enable them to avoid the sixty-vote obstacle in the Senate—reconciliation, an optional deficit control step in the congressional budget process laid out in the Congressional Budget Act of 1974." This allowed them to limit the types of amendments, circumvent the traditional supermajority requirements, and close debate with a simple majority after 20 hours, thus transforming it into a "major policy implementation tool."[106]

House Democrats were unwilling to completely surrender to reconciliation in passing healthcare legislation. This reluctance led to further procedural problems, but, eventually, the House Budget Committee crafted The Reconciliation Act of 2010 (House bill 4872). Its language was born of negotiations between White House officials and Democratic congressional leaders, again working outside of the traditional legislative process. "Negotiations continued throughout early March (2010) as the House leadership assembled the necessary votes in their chamber. At the same time, drafters sought an estimate from the CBO and the Joint Committee on Taxation on how much PPACA would cost. ... The CO published a cost estimate of the reconciliation bill as revised which came in under the budget target."[107]

The House was the first to vote. Debate was limited to two hours. On the evening of March 21, 2010, the Senate version of House bill 3590 passed the House. Previously approved by the Senate and sent for the president's signature, House bill 4872 passed soon after, and was sent to the Senate, which could not vote until the president signed 3590. The debate took place over two days, and 4872 was passed in the Senate on March 25, 2010.

For the third time in the history of modern healthcare policy, the absence of analysis and debate on significant and transforming legislation was simply amazing. This time, however, it was breathtaking because its aim was nothing less than redesigning the whole system, as the caption of Title III puts it, to "Improve the Quality and Efficiency of Health Care" for all Americans. Never mind that, during the preceding forty years, absolutely nothing federal or state agencies had done to control quality or costs worked.

The new legislation was not born of some definitive epiphany. Instead, it simply threw enormous sums of money at the problem, funding lots of "research" to allow staff and contractors to determine national priorities, to create numerous "demo" projects, and to pay incentives to providers to participate. Much of this was inserted into the legislation with the proviso that it would not be subject either to administrative or judicial review, and with very limited legislative review.

Instead of allowing market forces and consumers to determine how and at what price care should be provided, everything—from insurance provisions to delivery of care—was put under the direction, prerogative, and control of "the Secretary [of Health and Human Services]." The bureaucrats wanted it all, and Congress gave it to them.

Subtitle A under Title III makes it clear that the goal is "Transforming the Health Care Delivery System" through a "National Strategy to Improve Health Care Quality" entirely controlled by government regulators and bureaucrats. As explained in Chapter 4, the March 2010 MedPac Commission report stated this motive even clearer in its covering letter: "Reorganization of how care is delivered may be necessary for payment reform to work." Cost control now became the justification for delivering control of the healthcare system entirely into the hands of the administrative state—in direct contravention of the original Medicare statute. As the 2007 MedPac report had put it: "An important provision within Medicare's statute precludes the program from exercising any supervision or control over the practice of medicine."[108]

CHAPTER 6

The ACA Sinkhole

NEVER HAS MORE MONEY BEEN SPENT TO GET ABSOLUTELY NOTHING

The ACA legislation is a veritable grab bag.[109] There is something for everyone, including a huge hole for taxpayers. Random examples include $1.5 billion for grants relating to Indian Early Childhood programs, $400 million for grants to adult protective programs, $200 million for grants to employers for wellness programs, $900 million for centers of excellence devoted to depression, and hundreds of millions to fund training programs on ombudsmen improvement, surveyor abuse awareness, public health fellowships, and various clinical programs. The details are beyond the scope of this book, but catch-all diversity bespeaks a wish list rather than a strategic plan.

The ACA money was being scattered far and wide, the annual costs are hard to get a handle on because many items are open-ended, dependent on funding from other sources, and subject to further appropriations after a few years. Nevertheless, my own calculation of readily quantifiable additional direct federal outlays for Title II (Medicaid) and Title III (Medicare) appropriations as outlined in the original legislation is approximately $33 billion over the first ten years (2010-2019). The additional administrative overhead that accompanies all of this presents an even murkier picture. Indeed, we won't attempt to cut through the fog, but we can be certain that it adds untold billions to the $33 billion figure.

Nor will we address ACA insurance provisions, healthcare exchanges, Medicaid and CHIP expansion, and other costly aspects of the law, which in 2012 the non-partisan Congressional Budget Office (CBO) estimated would amount to an additional $1.76 trillion from 2012 to 2023. As of 2020, it has already mushroomed well beyond the CBO estimate because of basic cost overruns and the lack of implementation of the various taxes and penalties that were originally planned to pay for it. The insurance provisions have been the subject of endless political debate and many legislative actions over the years but are not pertinent to our purpose here, which is to expose the intentions of the law and its effect on the delivery of healthcare services.

SOME PRECURSORS

ACA was preceded by two other pieces of legislation. The first was the American Recovery and Reinvestment Act of August 2009, which allocated $1.2 billion for computerization—$598 million for 70 Health Information Technology Centers and $564 million for a Nationwide Health Information Network. The second was the Health Information Tech for Economic and Health Act (HITECH) of 2009, which allocated $27 billion to incentivize hospitals and physicians to computerize, adding billions more to fund assistance to and training of providers. Funds for computerization of long-term care facilities were left out of this legislation, so $67.5 million was allocated for this purpose at Section 2041 of the ACA.

In answer to MedPac's 2008 recommendations for "Reforming the Delivery System" and reorganizing the "health care system at a fundamental level," the ACA legislation (Title III, Part II, Sec. 3011) mandates: "The Secretary ... shall establish a national strategy to improve the delivery of health care services, patient health outcomes, and population health." The intention was to include "agency-specific strategic plans to achieve national priorities" and "strategies to align public and private payers" with these goals.

This is nothing other than euphemistic language for government control of an industry that currently commands almost 20 percent of our economy. It is the prelude to the eventual goal of single-payer, socialized medicine. With this purpose in mind, the authors of the legislation insert "The Secretary" approximately 3,000 times into the ACA text. A third of these references are dictates that the Secretary make the determinations, establish various programs and centers, conduct business, ensure program adequacy, provide reports, award grants, and establish the contracts necessary to carry out the larger mandate.

This chapter reviews how the ACA is quietly and discreetly aimed at accomplishing total control. The dimensions of this legislation are truly extraordinary, of a scope never encountered previously in this country. The aim is to lead us subtly down a path that cannot easily be reversed. Ultimately, the course will be headlong into massive industry consolidation and single-payer medicine. The timeframes are strung out; for achieving the objectives of this legislation will take some time. As former MedPac chairman Glenn Hackbarth wrote in the Executive Summary in the March 2010 MedPac Commission Report, "delivery system reforms ... will have to be investigated and successful models adopted on a broad scale. That is unlikely to happen in the near term."[110] Thus, the legislation allocated tremendous sums of money well into the future, earmarked for planning, developing standards, and implementing demo projects on a scale that will, over time, lead to radical and far-reaching changes in our system of delivering care. They will make it almost impossible to reverse course and return to a free-market solution.

THE CENTER FOR MEDICARE AND MEDICAID INNOVATION

The ACA legislation (Part III, Sec. 3021) added Section 1115A to Title XI of the Social Security Act, and established a new unit within CMS called the Center for Medicare and Medicaid Innovation (CMI), with an unending appropriation of $1 billion yearly, and except for Congressional activity reports, enjoying waiver authority over other requirements in the SSA, and an explicit exemption from administrative or judicial review of its activities. On the face of it, the mandate is to "test innovative payment and service delivery models to reduce program expenditures under the applicable titles (MR and MD), while preserving or enhancing the quality of care furnished to individuals under such titles."

But look closer, specifically at subsections (xi), (xiii), and (xviii) under (b) (2)(B). You will find a broader agenda, including "all-payer" payment reform and structural changes to "the full spectrum" of care delivery, as MedPac had been recommending. This level of funding—absent review—gives CMS free rein to maneuver the healthcare system as its officials see fit. Although CMS is required to file an annual report to Congress on these activities, the March 2018 GAO report titled "CMS Innovation Center: Model Implementation and Center Performance" clarified that Congress (Section 1115A) has "provided CMS with additional authority," including "expand[ing] the duration and scope of the models tested ... through rulemaking instead of needing the enactment of legislation," as traditionally required.[111]

Under Sections 3022, 3023, and 3024 the Center for Innovation was directed to implement three model programs proposed by MedPac in its June 2008 report, and discussed in Chapter 4: Accountable Care Organizations (ACOs), Bundled Payments for Episodes of Care, and Independence at Home (or medical home). What was not fully apparent in the earlier MedPac discussions was abundantly clear now. There was a huge bias toward hospital control of the integrated care that was being legislated. This bias was present even though, in the past, MedPac had cited concerns over hospital consolidation. For instance, in March of 2005, MedPac cited Federal Trade Commission (FTC) and Blue Cross Blue Shield (BCBS) complaints that industry consolidation forces private insurers to pay higher prices for hospital services, as the hospitals use their market power to negotiate higher prices. MedPac also found that when financial pressure diminished, as it would with consolidation, hospital costs grow faster.[112]

Despite these earlier expressed concerns, by March 2009, MedPac was looking for ways to justify the consolidation advocated in the model programs it was proposing. It stated that "consolidation could be beneficial if it reorganized the delivery system to make it more efficient. ... The Commission has recommended exploring forms of organization that would encourage collaboration between physicians and hospitals for care coordination and strengthen the role of primary care." MedPac continued: "the challenges facing Medicare require addressing the incentives and organization of the health care system at a fundamental level," and it tried to play down the degree to which industry consolidation affects costs, saying that it is an "additional" and "smaller" factor than other "disparate causes" such as the "constantly evolving" system, new technology, the nation's wealth, rising prices, health insurance impacts, and so on.[113]

But attempting to put a positive spin on a factor generally acknowledged and proved to have a negative impact is dangerous, and we have demonstrated—and will continue to demonstrate—how the consumers and taxpayers are being burned.

Section 3022, Accountable Care Organizations (ACOs), directs the Secretary to establish a "shared savings program" that "promotes accountability for a patient population and coordinates items and services under [Medicare] parts A and B." Only "groups of providers of services and suppliers meeting criteria specified by the Secretary may work together to manage and coordinate care." In describing what is necessary to be approved as an ACO, Section 3022 states that the organization "must have established a mechanism for shared governance," have a "formal legal structure" in place to accept liability for the care delivered across settings, have "a leadership and management structure that includes clinical and administrative systems," and have enough primary care physicians to serve a patient group of 5,000 lives. Section 3023 discusses bundling all services involved with a given hospitalization, including post-acute care, and that a formal "entity" must exist to receive the bundled payment for these services. Section 3024 likewise discusses the need for a common "legal strategy" for the various healthcare services offered so as to create a viable, authorized Independence at Home demonstration project. These directives thus soft pedaled vertical integration as well as horizontal consolidation. As a 2010 Merritt Hawkins white paper for the Physicians Foundation recognized, only organizations large enough to include physicians, hospitals, and other providers under one umbrella would be able to meet the specified legal criteria.[114]

The government's huge role in regulating and paying for care will draw providers toward these government-desired models for fear of losing market position and competitive advantage, including cozy relations with the regulators. The race to gain or maintain competitive advantage has fed acceptance of the ACO concept. A whole organization, the National Association of ACOs (NAACOS), has sprung up to (as their website proclaims) "foster growth of ACO models of care, ... participate with federal agencies in development and implementation of public policy,... and contribute to and shape policy agenda." NAACOS calls itself "THE voice of ACOs to CMS, the White House and on Capitol Hill."[115]

As of January 2018, NAACOS had "561 Medicare ACOs serving 12.3 million beneficiaries with hundreds more commercial and Medicaid ACOs serving millions of additional patients."[116] Yet, up to the time of the ACA legislation, similar projects were limited in scope and did "not present a precedent for future application." The current goal of this organization and the legislation it promotes is to expand and standardize the ACO concept, which will in turn lead to dangerous consolidation of market power which will be discussed further later.

RESULTS OF THE CENTER FOR INNOVATION DEMO PROJECTS

According to a March 2018 GAO Report to Congressional Requesters, by the end of 2016, which is the latest period for which data on resources used was available, the Center for Innovation had obligated $5.6 billion of its $10 billion appropriation for fiscal years 2011 to 2019 in order to implement 17 new demo models and assume responsibility for 20 more projects already started by CMS before the center was inaugurated. Some of these projects could also receive additional funding from the Medicare Trust Fund, and thus augment the center's budget. In accordance with the lack of oversight established by Congress, this GAO report was limited to examining payments made to the center, the use of funds, and center's assessment of its own performance. The center is free to pursue its own directions as long as they fit into the broad parameters outlined in the legislation, no matter what harm it could inflict on the industry. As of Sept. 30, 2017, it had a staff of 617 to carry out its programs.[117]

The latest complete data regarding the center's evaluation of its own progress is from 2015. Nothing is available for 2017 and 2018. The implementation of two more demo projects was planned for 2018, as of the date of the 2018 GAO report. In addition, 10 of the 37 projects implemented had been concluded. As of 2017, all demo participants are to be voluntary. Funding of models that had already been implemented ranged from $8.4 million to $967 million each. The GAO stated that "The Innovation Center has used the results from model evaluations to generate ideas for new models. For some of the early implemented models, evaluation results showed reduced spending and maintained or improved quality of care, but also identified model design limitations that could affect those results."[118] To be recertified for expansion, the model must adequately demonstrate reduced Medicare spending while maintaining or improving quality of care. The only two programs recertified were the Pioneer ACO and a Diabetes Prevention Program run by the YMCA.

The ACO Demo Program

The GAO reported that despite the $710.8 million obligated for these projects through 2016, CMS reported "mixed results" regarding the success of its ACO initiatives, especially in the area of shared savings. The report added, however, that CMS expected results to improve as the ACOs gained more experience with the program and moved to recertify the projects based on these expectations.[119]

The June 2018 MedPac report identified one demo, the Pioneer ACOs, as performing better than others and pointed out that Pioneer had enlisted organizations with some prior experience in risk-taking. However, MedPac also stated that, overall, the risk-taking groups produced "small savings." In fact, they were less than 1% against the benchmark, and this razor-thin savings was due to "reductions in the use of post-acute care and not from reductions in inpatient care." The most advanced group of providers, the NextGen ACOs, realized only a 0.2% net savings, even though participants could designate the level of risk-taking desired, provide incentives to beneficiaries to use their network, and use Medicare program waivers to avoid three-day hospital stays before being able to qualify for skilled nursing benefits.[120]

The June 2018 MedPac report also voiced concerns about the continued viability of hospital participation as ACOs because their leading motives, to fill beds and increase revenue, conflicted with ACO cost-reduction goals. The report observed that, to date, "ACOs have not caused a large reduction in inpatient admissions, despite rhetoric to the contrary." In addition, as of June 2018, of the 656 ACOs, only 55 participated as "advanced model" ACOs, accepting two-sided (profit and loss) risk. Thus, although the hospitals clearly enjoy the opportunity to use the government models as an excuse to expand their reach and dominate the provision of care in their regions, it does not appear that they want to put themselves at risk for acute care, let alone post-acute or chronic care management. MedPac temporized, stating that, at this late date, the program "continues to evolve."[121]

Recent ACO models aim at ensuring that both the provider and the payer share financial risk in providing care, while also increasing flexibility. The Medicare Access and CHIP Reauthorization Act (MACRA) of 2015 provided stronger incentive for providers to move into Alternative Payment Models (APMs). The ACO Improvement Act of 2017 allowed CMS to make ACO pilot programs permanent if they were determined to be successful. The Bipartisan Budget Act of 2018 added the ability of the ACO plan participants to include more non-medical incentives for high-risk individuals, to use telehealth (digital telecommunication technologies in place of in-person clinician contact), and to have more options in choosing program participants. Added incentives included paying beneficiaries up to $20 for each qualifying primary care visit with a provider in the ACO's network—outlays that were not to be charged against the ACO in calculating net savings. The 2018 act also extended the Independence at Home project to 15,000 lives, gave it another year to prove savings, and created more studies to determine long-term risk factors for chronic conditions.

The result? It appears that the hospitals still do not want to accept the levels of risk the program is ultimately seeking.

Although both the GAO and MedPac assessed that, overall, quality is being maintained or improving, this is generally true across all the programs and is not directly related to provisions of the 2018 legislation. Indeed, it would be expected that providers who voluntarily participate in a demo that offers incentives to produce results would reach the goals set.

The June 2018 MedPac report summed up ACO performance to date as demonstrating only slightly greater savings relative to what Medicare (FFS) spending would have been without ACOs. Consistent with this evaluation, the report stated that ACOs have "not caused a large reduction in inpatient admissions, despite rhetoric to the contrary."[122] Looking ahead, then, expectations should be very low for the redesigned ACO program CMS announced in December 2018, a program intended to lure more ACO participation with promises of greater shared savings and intended to induce participating institutions to assume even higher levels of risk, and sooner—that is, upon entering the program. Unobtainable savings goals and levels of risk assumption that are not desired should drastically limit participation in the program.

The Bundled Payments Demo

The Bundled Payment demo project offers participants an array of model choices, types of clinical episodes, episode characteristics, program rule waivers, and protective financial arrangements with other parties. This enormous range of flexibility differs so sharply from conditions in the real world as to disqualify all results from meaningful application.

In its third report to CMS, as revised in October 2018, The Lewin Group came to the same conclusion, stating that study participants responded to the financial incentives offered, but noted:

> There are relatively few instances in which these responses significantly changed key outcomes. Because of the vast range of situations encompassed under the initiative, including the selective and heterogeneous group of participants, and the limited and varied experience of participants, it is challenging to reach conclusions about the overall impact of BPCI. It is also important to keep in mind that the kind of changes envisioned under the initiative often need to occur within complex organizations and require collaboration across organizations that may have differing objectives.

The Lewin Group report pointed out further that "changes in care have not been correlated" with financial incentives and "there have not been systematic improvements as might be expected with incentives to coordinate care across an episode."[123] Yet, the project is to live on. Despite the $159.7 million that the GAO noted had been obligated for this project through 2016, and the fact that the fifth and final Lewin Group report stated "Medicare spending was higher under the initiative relative to what would have been spent," and "additional research is needed to calibrate what type and level of financial rewards are required to entice participants into reducing episode payments without completely offsetting those lower payments," the CMI nevertheless simply moved on into the "advanced" model, using "several key changes designed to help ensure net Medicare savings."[124]

The Independence at Home Demo

The November 2018 HHS report to Congress revealed that there were eighteen primary care practices participating in the demo. All had previous experience in specialized home-based care, thereby effectively undercutting the demo by demonstrating the ability of the market to experiment and develop new models on its own, independent of government, in search of better quality and more efficient care. Nevertheless, HHS reported that, after three years of the demo, it found only "indications that the demonstration may have reduced total Medicare expenditures and inpatient hospital expenditures" and if so, the reductions were estimated to be so "small" that they were "not statistically significant." The results were therefore deemed inconclusive. Yet, again, the report discussed continuing the demonstration for additional years in an attempt to "see stronger results,"[125] even though, as the GAO report notes, $64.2 million had already been allocated through 2016.[126] In effect, the report seemed to be arguing not for acting in response to the demo results (or non-results) but for testing until something that might be construed as the desired results had been achieved.

The Medicaid Home Health Demo

This demo is similar to the medical home, or Independence at Home, model just discussed—but, as stated in the May 2018 HHS report to Congress, with a "focus on high-need, high-cost Medicaid populations with chronic conditions" and "greater emphasis on coordinated care," which program creators considered a "critical element for integrating physical and behavioral health care services and linking patients with nonclinical services." As of December 2017, there were 32 programs implemented in 21 states, which were in addition to the many other programs initiated over decades by states attempting to manage this same population. In fact, the demos in most of the 21 states were "built on pre-existing structures and care coordination programs." CMS also works "collaboratively with each state to provide technical assistance" and actually requires states to seek CMS advice and consultation to fine-tune their programs and improve results.[127]

The report only covered results obtained from the first 13 programs in the first 11 states to launch these newest coordinated care projects. CMS stated that the programs in this demo "suggest the potential for improvements in care management," however it also added that it was "important to note the limitations to these findings" for it can be "very difficult ... to separate health home-specific effects from the effects of other initiative and delivery system changes occurring at the same time." CMS also stated that "results available to date are from periods early in the programs when implementation was far from complete."[128] The June 2018 MedPac report puts it more succinctly and realistically. Evaluations of the demonstration are taking longer to complete than expected. Furthermore, participation was lower than expected, for many (25%) of the enrollees satisfied with their previous care dropped out, so did those who were sicker. There was also broad agreement that the program was difficult to implement, and eighteen of sixty-eight demo participants dropped out.[129]

The GAO report noted that a staggering $769.9 million had been allocated for this program through 2022. It is important to note that by the time of these reports, the bulk of this money has been spent, and CMS has not been able to produce any more concrete results for the taxpayers, yet expects them to hang in there and let the agency spend more of their money on what it happens to somehow consider as indications that the demo "shows promise as a tool for improving care and achieving cost savings."[130]

Other Major Projects Being Funded by the Center

- $143.5 million obligated through 2020 to test partnerships between independent contractors and SNFs to try and reduce hospitalizations for MR/MD beneficiaries.[131]

- $338.7 million obligated through 2019 to push clinical practices "from volume to value-based delivery systems."[132]

- $559.4 million obligated through 2016 to fund contractors to test whether a coordinated, national collaborative for systematically spreading known best practices in patient safety could make acute care hospitals safer, more reliable, and less costly.[133]

- $2.066 billion obligated through 2018 to provide funding to states and local governments to also test new care delivery and payment models.[134]

The lack of review on these CMI projects, despite the billions of dollars in spending enumerated above, is truly shocking. What is far worse, is that similar projects have been ongoing for decades without success, and no evidence of any current breakthroughs have been published or seen in the industry. In truth, the Center has no concrete evidence that any demo project was properly conceived or achieved any outcome commensurate with the time and money spent, and cannot justify the possible negative effects on the structure of the industry. Thus, the Center has no reason to continue and every reason to discontinue spending. It is time for Congress to intervene. The couple of relatively minor projects that show potential, albeit weakly, are very narrowly constructed and therefore of little, perhaps negligible, consequence. As the *Wall Street Journal* article on what it costs to do a knee operation illustrates, market pressure will achieve the desired results much more efficiently.[135]

THE CENTER FOR HEALTHCARE QUALITY IMPROVEMENT

In addition to creating the Center for Innovation, the ACA legislation (Part III, Subtitle F, Sec. 3501) amended Section 3013 of Part D of Title IX of the Public Health Service Act (PL 78-410 [1944]). Section 933, titled "Health Care Delivery System Research," provided initial funding of $20 million to "enable" the Director of the Center for Healthcare Quality Improvement within the CMS Agency for Healthcare Research and Quality to "identify, develop, evaluate, disseminate, and provide training in innovative methodologies and strategies for quality improvement practices in the delivery of health care services that represent best practices," including "changes in processes of care and the redesign of systems used by providers that will reliably result in intended health outcomes." The Director was further authorized to identify providers that "(A) deliver consistently high-quality, efficient healthcare services (as determined by the Secretary), and (B) employ best practices that are adaptable," and to gather research about "what strategies and methodologies are most effective." The Director was to take this acquired knowledge and "facilitate adoption of best practices," and "where applicable, assist ... providers across the continuum of care ... in improving the care and patient health outcomes." Section 934 authorized technical assistance grants for providers trying to implement these best practices.

In other words, the bureaucrats were empowered to determine best practices, learning from those considered the best in the industry, and instead of allowing poor-performing providers to fail, as would happen in a normal marketplace, Congress for some reason opted to use taxpayer money to try to teach them and thereby keep them in business, a concept at odds with any rational thought, and which continues to frustrate the taxpayers.

The Patient Centered Outcomes Research Institute

One of the most peculiar provisions of the ACA (Sec. 6301) is the establishment of a non-profit organization called the Patient-Centered Outcomes Research Institute (PCORI). As such, it is neither an agency nor an establishment of the United States Government, yet its funding for ten years (2011-2019) comes from the U.S. Treasury and fees levied on insurance plans.

The $3.4 billion appropriation to fund an agency that did not previously exist and is outside of normal government controls is absolutely astounding. The institute is free to develop its own research priorities and agenda without having to adhere to the national priorities that the Secretary must establish under the ACA. Moreover, it has the resources of the Assistant Secretary for Planning and Evaluation (ASPE) for assistance, yet the ASPE already advises the Secretary on policy development, coordinates the Department's evaluation, research, and demonstration activities, and conducts research and evaluation studies.

The stated purpose of the institute is to "assist patients, clinicians, purchasers, and policy makers in making informed health decisions by advancing the quality and relevance of evidence concerning how diseases, disorders, etc. can effectively and appropriately be prevented, diagnosed, treated and managed through (clinical effectiveness) research, evidence synthesis and dissemination." Yet, CMS has its own Agency for Healthcare Quality and Research and a newly created Center for Medicare and Medicaid Innovation to provide these very same functions. The mandate for the Agency for Healthcare Quality and Research was discussed earlier, and, as mentioned, one of the projects the Center for Innovation established involves funding other contractors—in the amount of $559.4 million—to test whether a coordinated, national collaborative for systematically disseminating known best practices in patient safety could make acute care hospitals safer, more reliable, and less costly. In addition, there are at least two other massive, long-established government agencies—the National Institutes of Health (NIH) and the Centers for Disease Control and Prevention (CDC)—and countless other privately and publicly funded research projects with mandates for the same type of research.

The only required review of the new institute's activity is to be done every *fifth* year by the GAO, which is charged simply with determining whether the institute's work product appears objective, credible, and produced in a manner consistent with the requirements of the legislation.

The first GAO review, in March of 2018, stated that, of the 543 research projects the institute awarded through 2017, only 53 had been completed because nearly two-thirds of the funds committed ... were awarded in fiscal years 2015-2017, and the research process established by PCORI can take as long as 6 years to complete. In effect, the Institute had already spent or committed approximately $2,330,000,000 without any evaluation of its activities! Of this, it had spent $310 million on program and administrative support services, and committed about $1.6 billion in research awards, as well as $325 million to build capacity to use existing health data for research.[136]

HHS had received $448 million from its mandated 20% allocation of PCORI's funding, and it had obligated $260 million, or 58%, of the funds for dissemination and implementation of research produced by the institute. However, the report noted that since "most PCORI-funded [research] had not yet been completed due to the time needed to conduct this research, HHS efforts focused instead on the dissemination and implementation of [research] funded by other federal entities," including those mentioned above. On the face of it, this new non-profit organization hardly seems necessary.

The GAO stated that of the five PCORI submissions HHS (AHRQ) considered for publication during 2017, only one was under consideration for implementation as of December 2017. Two PCORI submissions were rejected—one because of insufficient impact and the other because of challenges in implementation feasibility. Two other submissions were still under review.

Obviously, this is not a good track record for the applicability of PCORI's research, which only made up 13% of the submissions to HHS to begin with. Little wonder that the GAO stated that PCORI had only "begun efforts to track implementation, such as the number of its findings published in peer-reviewed journals, and the use of its findings in clinical care."[137] However, when research projects take six years or more to complete and then the data must be synthesized for use by providers or the public, the question becomes: How current and useful is the substantially aged information? The world moves on, overtaking the research and its consumers.

The GAO report shows annual institute funding increasing from $50 million in 2010 to $466,085,000 in 2017. It ended 2017 with $1,033.061 billion in assets because it took in far more funding than it could commit. Yet it also had $92,735,675 in liabilities for contracts granted. The funding for 2017 consisted of $105 million from the Hospital Insurance Funds, $235.4 million from fees on insurance plans, $120M from General Fund appropriations (this is net of the $30 million to HHS), and $5.7 million in interest income. The report states: "By the end of fiscal year 2024, PCORI projects to have spent a total of almost $3.3 billion, which reflects its projected Trust Fund revenue through fiscal year 2019 plus interest income."[138] In other words, funding will have ended in 2019 but operations are projected to continue through 2024. What is planned for this organization and its 617 employees (per the 2018 GAO report) in 2024 is not discussed, but it is doubtful that it will simply be disbanded.

To sum up, one of the most incredibly bizarre aspects of the ACA is that Congress handed billions of dollars to a non-profit organization, that had to be created de novo, to fund what appears to be unnecessary, duplicative, and dilatory research as it sees fit—all without proper review or coordination of activities.

QUALITY MEASURES

The ACA legislation included a minimum of $615 million to continue to develop quality measures. Under Section 2701, Medicaid Quality Measures, the Secretary was allocated $240 million and directed to identify and publish a recommended core set of health quality measures for Medicaid-eligible adults and use them to establish a Medicaid Quality Measurement Program. Under Section 3013, the Secretary was allocated another $375 million to identify the need for improvement in existing quality measures consistent with the national strategy for use in federal health programs. The section also requires the Secretary to develop and periodically update provider-level outcome measures for hospitals and physicians, as well as other providers. All of this follows decades and billions of wasted taxpayer funds trying to define various aspects of service quality and how to rate and pay providers. Market studies indicate that the public ignores the government data and provider ratings, substituting for these its own criteria. Examples of this are found in the June 2018 MedPac report. The following occur in a discussion of what CMS defines as quality "post-acute care" (PAC) providers:

- "Medicare has developed consumer-oriented websites that provide information on the quality of SNFs and HHAs, but many studies have concluded that these efforts have not significantly increased the use of higher quality PAC providers."

- "For example, over 94 percent of beneficiaries who used HHA or SNF services had at least one provider within a 15-mile radius that had higher performance on a composite quality indicator than the provider they selected."[139]

- "The evidence suggests that Medicare's Nursing Home Compare and Home Health Compare data have minimal impact in motivating beneficiaries to choose higher quality providers."

- "One study found that most SNF patients did not appear to select higher quality providers after the Medicare.gov data were released to consumers, while another found that the data had a small impact (an increase of less than 1 percent of a facility's volume) when there was a large difference in the quality of available providers (Werner et al. 2012, Werner et al. 2011). A review of the impact of the HHA data available through Medicare.gov also found minimal impact."

- "A 2004 survey of [hospital] discharge planners found that, while 63 percent of planners were aware of the PAC quality data that Medicare makes available, only 38 percent reported using it (Castle 2009)."

- "In practice, beneficiaries report soliciting the views of physicians, family members, or other associates to recommend a PAC provider (Advisory Board Company 2016, Harris and Beeuwkes-Buntin 2008, Shugarman and Brown 2006). ... Beneficiaries generally view this information as more valuable than comparative quality data available through sources like Medicare.gov (Advisory Board Company 2016, Harris and Beeuwkes Buntin 2008, Sefcik et al. 2016)."[140]

Note the condescending attitudes reflected in these statements. Neither the agencies nor the commission yields an inch to the consumer's ability to judge service quality or rate providers. The bureaucrats simply refuse to give up control. For example, in discussing the possibility of allowing hospitals to come up with their own quality ratings on PAC providers, the MedPac committee acknowledges that "beneficiaries would receive recommendations that reflect quality of PAC care in the market," but since that could result in "multiple definitions [of quality] across hospitals," there would be a need for "CMS approval of individual hospitals' criteria and monitoring of proper application."[141]

Here are more examples, these from discussions concerning judging quality in the acute setting:

- "Over the past several years, the Commission has expressed concern that Medicare's quality measurement programs are "overbuilt," relying on too many clinical process measures that are, at best, weakly correlated with health outcomes of importance to beneficiaries and the program."[142]

- "Too many overlapping hospital quality payment and reporting programs create unneeded complexity for hospitals and the Medicare program. All-condition measures are more appropriate to measure the performance of hospitals. ... Some of the programs score hospitals using "tournament models" rather than "clear, absolute, and prospectively set performance targets."[143]

- "Ideally, Congress could redesign the multiple hospital quality payment programs under a single quality payment program that would be patient oriented, encourage coordination across providers and time, and promote change in the delivery system. Although CMS likely has the authority to make some of the suggested changes ... without congressional action (e.g., improving public reporting), other key reforms would require statutory changes."[144]

- In June of 2014 and 2015 the committee was suggesting an alternative Medicare quality incentive program that "would use a small set of outcomes, patient experience, and value measures to assess the quality of care across different populations," and then link these performance measures to payment.[145]

Note how complex the matter becomes when attempting to tie payment to quality measures. Also note the level of responsibility that falls on Congress in these matters. Congress is called upon far too often to legislate specific demo programs and payment methods. It is time that Congress and the agencies devote their energies to aspects of health care they more fully understand, such as benefits or program entitlements, and let the marketplace determine the services, quality, and price desired—and thus, ultimately, who will survive as providers.

In a freely competitive environment, quality providers would be constantly innovating and improving the cost effectiveness and quality of their services or products, and the consumers would be the ultimate decision makers. Quality should never be considered a static concept, which can be chiseled for all time into legislation or regulation. By the time the research is done, models developed, demos completed, and laws and regulations published, the state of knowledge and technology, and concepts for service delivery will likely have substantially changed. And for the sake of the state of the art and science of healthcare, thank goodness for that.

If the bureaucrats would eliminate barriers to entry, allow quality providers to flourish, and new ideas to proliferate as happens in any other marketplace, quality and price would be determined very efficiently, and the consumer would be much better off. In a marketplace where everything is centrally "administered," administrators must determine standards of operation and proper indicators of value, what it should cost to deliver the service at that value, and be constantly trying to hold the provider responsible for missing the mark. Otherwise, obtaining value-based purchasing is impossible. As presently constituted, it *is* impossible. The system is characterized by demo projects, incentives, takebacks, and so on instead of letting the consumers and competition figure it all out in real time in the real world. The administrators must make the market, and hope they are right, or tremendous harm can be done. We have now had fifty years of tremendous harm. It is time for change.

THE BUREAUCRATIC MINDSET: WE NEED THEIR HELP

Beneficiaries should not need help identifying quality providers. What they need is to get rid of the regulations that disrupt proper functioning, such as those that interfere with letting hospital discharge planners do their job properly:

- "The Improving Medicare Post-Acute Care Transformation Act of 2014 requires hospitals to include quality data when informing beneficiaries about their options, but CMS has yet to finalize the regulations implementing this requirement."

- "Helping beneficiaries to identify better quality PAC providers should be a goal in a reformed discharge planning process, and authorizing hospital discharge planners to recommend specific higher quality PAC providers would further this goal."

- "In most reform models, CMS has not changed or waived any existing discharge planning requirements, and hospitals continue to be subject to the current regulations."[146]

Note the unintended irony of the statements that follow. The hospitals would have the "freedom" to establish their own criteria, yet must be "consistent in approach," using established, transparent quality standards, while being "responsible" to the regulators. The regulators are not about to stop controlling (establishing and enforcing) quality standards and the industry.

- "Under a flexible approach, hospitals would be responsible for defining the criteria they would use to identify higher quality PAC providers. A hospital would be responsible for selecting quality measures, collecting data from PAC providers, and setting the performance levels that PAC providers would have to meet to be recommended by the hospital."

- "The advantage of this approach is that it provides hospitals with the freedom to establish the criteria that they believe best reflect the needs of their patients and to tailor those criteria to the available supply of providers. Some hospitals have conducted similar processes to identify PAC referral partners for ACOs and bundled payment initiatives, for instance."

- However, several design decisions would need to be resolved. "First, a consistent approach to identifying better quality PAC providers would be needed, and quality standards would need to be transparent for PAC providers and beneficiaries." Secondly, Medicare discharge planning rules do not permit them to recommend specific PAC providers."[147]

CHAPTER 7

The Current State of Affairs

HOPELESSLY LOST

It is now a decade since the ACA legislation was passed. We have spent the billions in additional dollars it authorized for greatly expanded demonstration projects and research aimed at fundamentally changing our system. Chapter 6 illustrated how poorly the demonstration and research programs have fared. The Secretary of Health and Human Services was handed massive new responsibilities under the ACA while continuing to manage the current system. In its March 2019 report, MedPAC labeled managing the current system nothing more than an "interim responsibility."[148] Thus, despite the dollars spent these last ten years, and the preceding forty years, in vain pursuit of viable fundamental system change, this bureaucratic goal is still on the table. It is to be accomplished through the same means that produced nothing but failure: either more demonstration programs or more putative "improvements" to the current system or both. It appears to be both.

No matter what methods are used, Medicare has the heft to profoundly change the industry for better or worse, producing effects both intended and unintended.

In this chapter, I present a few examples of the incredible absence of understanding still on display from bureaucrats who persist in attempting to manage the "current" system, producing staggering costs to taxpayer and patient alike as the years roll by, consumed with discussion of policy and the making of arbitrary pricing decisions but coming no closer to the goal of value-based care. In the next chapter, I will go on to consider how pricing policies and the ACA demonstration projects have led to the current phenomenal level of industry consolidation by hospital systems nationwide.

The size and scope of the Medicare program and the influence on other programs are profound, especially within the current regulatory environment. Policy decisions based on theoretical and unproven concepts can be extremely dangerous. Demo projects, pricing policies, and the anticipation thereof may cause providers to move in directions solely to preserve or gain competitive advantage. This in turn may well produce unintended consequences and create permanent damage to the structure of a market forced to endure the real-world testing of ill-conceived legislative and administrative ideas.

ACUTE CARE

The examples discussed in Chapter 1 illustrating the lack of in-house knowledge to enable hospital systems to adequately price their own services proves the inadequacy of Medicare cost reports to provide reliable guidance for the bureaucrats charged with pricing these services. Worse still, hospitals are at the very top of the service triangle, leaving no alternative providers from which to obtain acute care and with which costs might be compared. Thus, MedPac faces significant obstacles in attempting to fulfill its mandate to determine whether hospital rates are reasonable or not. The March 2018 MedPac report noted that the commission uses four "indicators" to assess payment adequacy: patient access, quality levels, industry access to capital, and the relationship of payments to costs (gross profit margins) for "both average and relatively efficient hospitals."[149] Lately, MedPac has come to judge that these indicators demonstrate that Medicare rates are adequate. This determination, however, is based on the current marketplace structure, and the commission has no way of determining what rates would be charged in a fully competitive marketplace. The next chapter will discuss the many indicators suggesting that, as a whole, rates are far too high and rapidly leading to a hyper-consolidated monopolistic industry, which can only mean less choice and higher prices for taxpayer and healthcare consumer alike.

The March 2019 report stated that there are three current hospital quality incentive programs besides the Hospital Value-Based Purchasing Program, and noted that the commission "has several concerns about the design of these programs." Chief among them are that the programs create needless complexity, include process measures that are not consistently reported or tied to outcomes, and use scoring that is not focused on "clear, absolute, and prospectively set system of targets."[150] In June 2018, MedPac had examined the potential to create a single outcome-focused, quality-based payment program, and recommended to Congress that it be used to replace the current programs.[151]

POST-ACUTE CARE (PAC)

Although in general there is no typical competitive marketplace in post-acute care, there are various categories of service providers that were defined by the regulators over fifty years ago. Unfortunately, the needs of the marketplace and service delivery mechanisms were not fully understood then, and they are still not today. This presents a significant problem for the rate setters, who want to provide services in the most efficient setting but feel obligated to recognize the cost structures of operating these various organizations, much of which is dictated by government regulation.

The problem was recognized in the March 2018 MedPAC report which stated, "PAC [post-acute care] presents particular challenges in establishing accurate and equitable payments because it is not always clear whether the beneficiary requires PAC and, if so, which setting is best suited to the patient's care needs or how much care would yield the best outcome." The commission continued, noting that it has "previously discussed the challenges to increasing the accuracy of Medicare's payments and overcoming the shortcomings of the separate FFS payment systems for PAC. Over more than a decade, the Commission has worked extensively on PAC payment reform, pushing for closer alignment of costs and payments and more equitable payments across different types of patients."[152]

MedPac goes on to enumerate more of the "challenges" to creating accurate Medicare payments:

- "For years, the Commission has raised concerns that the PAC PPSs (prospective payment systems) encourage providers to favor treating some types of patients over others." Currently, there are "distortions in the SNF and HHA PPSs that encourage providers to furnish services of questionable value and advantage providers that avoid medically complex patients."[153]

- "There are few evidence-based guidelines for PAC, ... PAC placement decisions often reflect nonclinical factors, such as local practice patterns,

PAC availability in a market, the proximity to a beneficiary's home, patient and family preferences, and financial relationships between the referring hospital and the PAC provider—but not necessarily where the patient would receive the best care. Given these factors, it is not surprising that per capita Medicare spending varies more for PAC than for any other service (Medicare Payment Advisory Commission 2017b). Across the four PAC settings, Medicare requires providers to use different patient assessment tools, which undermines the program's ability to compare on a risk-adjusted basis the patients admitted, the cost of care, and the outcomes patients achieve. Finally, though similar beneficiaries can be treated in the four settings, Medicare uses separate payment systems for each that can result in considerably different payments for comparable conditions. These factors led the Congress to include mandated studies of a unified payment system in the Improving Medicare Post Acute Care Transformation Act of 2014 (IMPACT)."[154]

- "Since 1999, the Commission has called for a variety of quality initiatives, including the collection of uniform patient assessment information, the reporting of outcome-based quality measures that focus on the key goals of PAC, and the implementation of value-based purchasing policies. ... In 2016, in response to a congressional mandate (The Improving Medicare Post-Acute Care Transformation Act (IMPACT) of 2014), the Commission recommended design features of a unified payment system to be used in the four PAC settings to ... replace the four independent PPSs in use today." Although "On the quality front, there has been progress on defining common outcome measures across PAC providers and establishing value-based purchasing policies for HHAs (on a demonstration basis) and for SNFs, ... the Commission is increasingly concerned that trends in some provider-reported quality measures raise questions about the accuracy and reliability of this information. The Commission has work underway to examine the accuracy of the patient assessment–based quality measures."[155]

- "Distortions encouraged by the payment systems have resulted in practice patterns that do not reflect efficient care. In contrast to traditional FFS, there is some evidence that Medicare Advantage plans and providers participating in alternative payment models (such as accountable care organizations and bundled payment initiatives) refer fewer patients to PAC, use lower cost PAC settings, and, in the case of SNFs, have shorter and less therapy-intensive stays—without appearing to harm patient outcomes (Colla et al. 2016, Dummit et al. 2016, Huckfeldt et al. 2017, McWilliams et al. 2016, Winblad et al. 2017). ... In addition to providers' financial incentives created by the PPS's current designs, specific concerns about PAC have framed the Commission's discussions of the need to reform the way Medicare pays for this care."[156]

- "Specifically, the skilled nursing facility (SNF) prospective payment system (PPS) favors treating rehabilitation over medically complex patients, encourages providers to furnish therapy unrelated to a patient's condition, and poorly targets payments for patients requiring high-cost non-therapy ancillary services (such as expensive antibiotics). The home health agency (HHA) PPS encourages agencies to provide therapy services, provide enough visits to avoid short-stay payments, and—in select states with value-based purchasing in place—code frailty to increase payments. The inpatient rehabilitation facility (IRF) PPS appears to encourage some providers to admit certain types of patients and code clinical conditions and impairments in a way that raises payments relative to the cost of care. The long-term care hospital (LTCH) PPS encourages providers to extend the duration of stays to qualify for full payment, rather than a lesser short-stay payment. Partly reflecting differences in providers' practices, the financial performance of providers differs widely."[157]

- "The Commission recommended redesigns of the SNF (in 2008) and HHA payment systems (in 2011) that would base payments on patient characteristics such as diagnoses, comorbidities, and impairments, not the amount of therapy provided (Medicare Payment Advisory Commission 2011, Medicare Payment Advisory Commission 2008). The proposed changes would generally increase payments for medically complex care and decrease payments for rehabilitation care that is unrelated to a patient's characteristics."[158]

Skilled Nursing Facilities (SNFs)

In its March 2002 report, MedPac stated that "Medicare's payment policy for skilled nursing facility services has been caught in an action-reaction cycle over the past serval years. ... The classification system upon which the PPS is based is inadequate."[159]

The March 30, 2019 report stated that "CMS's work on alternative designs for the SNF PPS began 13 years ago in response to a legislative requirement (the Medicare, Medicaid, and SCHIP Benefits Improvement and Protection Act of 2000) to conduct research on potential refinements of the SNF PPS." The report noted that the value-based purchasing policy for SNFs began in October of 2018, but is only based on one factor, the percentage of hospital readmissions in the first 30 days. Two percent of payments are withheld from facilities until results are calculated, and only 25% of the facilities have received that withheld 2%. Thus, one may easily question the applicability of this factor to judge value.[160]

Home Health Agencies (HHAs)

"Policymakers have long struggled to define the role of the home health benefit in Medicare (Benjamin 1993)." The benefits are broad, guidelines are not often followed, and fraud and abuse are continuing challenges. Unlike the requirements for SNF eligibility, no hospital stay or co-pay is required, and the patient can easily get recertified for multiple 60 day episodes. "Between 1990 and 1995, the number of annual users rose by 75 percent, and the number of visits more than tripled to about 250 million a year. Spending increased more than fourfold between 1990 and 1995, from $3.7 billion to $15.4 billion. As the rates of use and the duration of home health spells grew, there was concern that the benefit was serving more as a long-term care benefit. (Government Accountability Office 1996). Further, many of the services provided were believed to be improper." After getting more restrictive on recertifications between 1997 and 2000, payments decreased 52%, and the number of home care agencies decreased 31%.[161]

In the March 2002 report, MedPac noted that the home health services "sector has seen massive swings in spending over the past few years. Although we do not yet have any cost data for the period since the PPS ... was put in place, the absence of clear evidence from other indicators of disparity between payments and costs in the sector leads us to conclude that the payment base as of 2002 is adequate." However, in March 2019, the MedPac report stated that "between 2002 and 2016, spending increased by over 88 percent. For more than a decade, payments under the home health prospective payment system (PPS) have consistently and substantially exceeded costs."[162]

With PPS, the mix of services changed from primarily aides, to nursing and therapy. Physical therapy grew to represent 39% of the home visits in 2016. In the commission's view, the PPS rates were not only established too high, but overpaid: "CMS currently makes a full 60-day payment for the 28 percent of episodes that are 30 days or shorter." Thus, due to mandates in the Bipartisan Budget Act of 2018, again, CMS is working on two new changes to correct this, but it is also planning to implement a new assessment system in 2020 called the Patient-Driven Groupings Model (PDGM), which "categorizes episodes into 432 payment groups," rather than the current 153 groups.[163]

In 2017, Medicare also initiated a value-based purchasing (VBP) demo for home health in nine states, which, as with a comparable hospital program, was to offer incentive bonuses for high performance. Quality was to be assessed by a composite of 20 measures of process, outcomes, and patient satisfaction. A CMS-contracted report "concluded that the impact of the VBP program on quality was mixed in 2017, the first year payments were adjusted under the program."[164]

In addition, the March 2019 Medpac report also stated that "the HHA value-based purchasing demonstration uses measures of function to calculate provider performance," noting, however, "it is important that it consistently and accurately reflects patients' levels of function" for it "creates incentives for providers to report it in ways that boost payments. ... we have become increasingly concerned about the validity and utility of provider-reported patient assessment information." The report continued: "The Commission is increasingly wary of the accuracy of the provider-reported patient assessment information. The Commission has work underway to assess these data. Although these data are important for measuring patient outcomes and establishing care plans, they may not be key to establishing accurate payments. Our initial work on a unified PAC PPS found that payments could be accurate without measures of patient function. The Commission will continue its work on design elements of a PAC PPS, including whether function is a necessary component of a case-mix system."[165]

Inpatient Rehabilitation Facilities (IRFs) and Long-term care Hospitals (LTCHs)

The March 2018 MedPac report stated that in 2016, 77% of the inpatient rehabilitation facilities were distinct units of acute care hospitals, with 50% of them operated by one national chain, at estimated profit margins around 41%. Likewise, two national chains were operating close to half of the long-term care hospitals. The need for these facilities was doubtful to begin with, and thus the commission continued to struggle over the appropriate levels of care and payment rates for these facilities. Since 2005, Congress had been adjusting the types of patients and payments these facilities were allowed.[166]

The report stated that, in March of 2014, the commission recommended the LTCH payment system be further reformed to differentiate between critically ill patients and those who were not critical. It also called for the system to establish "consistent payment between acute care hospitals and long-term care hospitals for certain categories of patients." In March of 2016, the commission recommended "changes to IRF rates as a short-term fix to better align payments with costs" and called for the "Secretary [to] improve program integrity" by reviewing medical records in conjunction with patient assessment data, to reassess the inter-rater reliability, and discern the accuracy of recorded patient acuity. Further, the commission recommended "elements of a unified PAC PPS that would make payments based on a patient's needs and characteristics, generally irrespective of the PAC entity that provided their care. … The Commission will continue to study other services that are provided in multiple sites of care to find additional services for which the principle of the same payment for the same service can be applied." In 2018, the commission continued to "assess aggregate trends in the quality" of the care rendered.[167]

PHYSICIAN PAYMENT

In its March 2002 report, MedPac stated:

> The current physician payment update formula, known as the sustainable growth rate (SGR) system, should be repealed. It causes large swings in updates from year to year that are unrelated to changes in the cost of furnishing physician services. … (p. xv) MedPac recognizes that one payment mechanism cannot simultaneously set individual prices accurately and control total spending on physician services delivered to Medicare beneficiaries. The SGR attempted to do so and failed.[168]

Sixteen years later, on March 2018, MedPac stated:

> The Commission remains concerned ["long-standing," (p. 199)] that evaluation and management (E&M) office visits, which make up a large share of the services provided by primary care clinicians and certain other specialties (e.g.,

psychiatry, endocrinology, and rheumatology), are underpriced in the fee schedule relative to other services, such as procedures. In addition, the nature of FFS payment allows some specialties to more easily increase the volume of services they provide (and therefore their revenue from Medicare). Such increases are less likely for other specialties, particularly those that spend most of their time providing labor-intensive E&M services. These factors contribute to an income disparity between primary care physicians and certain specialists. … Validation of the fee schedule's RVUs could help correct price inaccuracies and ensure that E&M office visits are not underpriced relative to other services. CMS has a statutory mandate and resources to validate RVUs, and the Commission has provided CMS with ideas for how to do so.[169]

"Recognizing that an enacted public policy is not fulfilling its intended goals and … calling for its elimination is complex," the March 2018 report continued:

For example, the sustainable growth rate (SGR) system, [begun in 1999, and] intended to limit growth in Medicare (physician) fee schedule spending to a formula based on GDP … was repeatedly overridden by the Congress between 2003 to 2014 and was not eliminated until the Medicare Access and CHIP Reauthorization Act of 2015 (MACRA). The Commission supports the elements of MACRA that repealed the SGR and encouraged comprehensive, patient-centered care delivery models such as advanced alternative payment models (A–APMs).

Notwithstanding …, the Commission has concluded that one part of MACRA, the Merit-based Incentive Payment System (MIPS), will not fulfill its goals and therefore should be eliminated. … The basic design of MIPS is fundamentally incompatible with the goals of a beneficiary-focused approach to quality measurement (p. xxvi). We recommend creating a new clinician value-based purchasing program [VVP] to take its place. … It is a core Commission principle for value-based purchasing programs that clinical outcomes, patient experience, and cost must be evaluated together and that these measures are dependent on the totality of the delivery system which produces them.[170]

A Parting Word on Undue Complexity: The Case of the Ambulatory Surgery Center

Medicare repeatedly proves itself capable of new heights of bureaucratic management complexity, which defy reason.

Procedure Codes

The March 2018 MedPac report stated that "Since 1982, Medicare has covered and paid for surgical procedures provided in ASCs [ambulatory surgical centers]." Within the ASC system, "Medicare covers surgical procedures represented by about 3,500 codes in the Healthcare Common Procedure Coding System (HCPCS). However, ASC volume for services covered under Medicare is concentrated in a relatively small number of HCPCS codes. For example, in 2016, 27 HCPCS codes accounted for 75 percent of the ASC volume for surgical services provided to Medicare beneficiaries."[171]

In its March 2009 report, MedPac noted that in 2008, CMS increased the number of surgical codes for ASCs by 32% even though it knew that 74% of the service volume was billed using 20 procedure codes.[172]

Payments

The March 2018 MedPac report states:

> For procedures performed in an ASC, Medicare makes two payments: one to the facility through the ASC payment system and the other to the physician for his or her professional services through the payment system for physicians and other health professionals, also known as the physician fee schedule (PFS).

> Medicare pays ASCs for a bundle of facility services— such as nursing, recovery care, anesthetics, and supplies— through a system that is primarily linked to the OPPS (outpatient prospective payment system), which Medicare uses to set payment rates for most services provided in HOPDs (Hospital Outpatient Departments). ... The ASC payment system is also partly linked to the PFS (prospective fee schedule).

> For most covered procedures, the ASC relative weight, which indicates a procedure's resource intensity relative to other procedures, is based on its relative weight under the OPPS. ...

> The ASC conversion factor is lower than the OPPS conversion factor because it started at a lower level in 2008 and has been updated since then at a lower rate than the OPPS conversion factor. ... In addition, since 2008, CMS has updated the ASC conversion factor based on the consumer price index for all urban consumers (CPI–U), whereas it has used the hospital market basket to update the OPPS conversion factor.

> We are concerned that the CPI–U may not reflect ASCs' cost structure ....

The Commission has recommended that ["Congress require" (March 2010 Med-Pac report, p. xvi)] CMS collect cost data from ASCs to identify an alternative price index that would be an appropriate proxy for ASC costs (Medicare Payment Advisory Commission 2010b). However, the ASC industry has opposed the collection of cost data for this purpose.

The 2010 report stated that in the past, the cost data came not from cost reports, but from surveys of costs that were done every 5 or 6 years, the latest being 2004. The March 2009 report also noted that only 20% of the typical ASC revenue came from Medicare, thus the hesitancy to be forced into the time and expense of mandated surveys or cost reports.

> CMS uses a different method from the one described above to determine payment rates for procedures that are [a] predominantly performed in physicians' offices and [b] were first covered under the ASC payment system in 2008 or later. Payment for these "office-based" procedures is the lesser of the amount derived from the standard ASC method or the practice expense portion of the PFS rate that applies when the service is provided in a physician's office (the non-facility practice expense, which covers the equipment, supplies, nonphysician staff, and overhead costs of a service). CMS set this limit on the rate for office-based procedures to prevent migration of these services from physicians' offices to ASCs for financial reasons.[173]

HOPD (hospital outpatient department) costs and efficiency compared to that of ASCs (ambulatory surgery centers)

The March 2019 MedPac report stated:

> Although we do not have recent ASC cost data that would allow us to quantify cost differences between settings, some evidence suggests that ASCs are a lower cost setting than HOPDs. The Government Accountability Office (GAO) compared ASC cost data from 2004 with HOPD costs and found that costs were, on average, lower in ASCs than in HOPDs (Government Accountability Office 2006). In addition, studies that used data from the National Survey of Ambulatory Surgery found that the average time for ambulatory surgical visits for Medicare patients was 25 percent to 39 percent lower in ASCs than HOPDs, which likely contributes to lower costs in ASCs (Hair et al. 2012, Munnich and Parente 2014). An additional study using data from a facility that has both an ASC and a hospital found that surgeries took 17 percent less time in the ASC. ...[174]

Yet in the next chapter we will see that as of 2019, HOPD rates are, in general, much higher than ASC rates.

Value-Based Purchasing

The March 2018 MedPac report stated:

> In 2012, the Commission recommended that the Congress authorize and CMS implement a value based purchasing (VBP) program for ambulatory surgical centers (ASCs). A VBP program would reward high-performing providers (Medicare Payment Advisory Commission 2012). ... The ASC VBP should include outcomes, patient experience, and value measures (a value measure would address services that are costly but of low value).[175]

Characteristically, the 2019 March MedPac notes that this has not been done: "Medicare payments to ASCs are not adjusted based on how they perform on quality measures, only on whether they report the measures. The Commission believes that high-performing ASCs should be rewarded and low-performing facilities should be penalized through the payment system."[176] However, CMS has more to worry about with how the rates are promulgated (which is discussed further in the next chapter) and eliminating the competitive advantages granted to HOPDs, than determining proper quality measures (which were discussed in the previous chapter) and being able to differentiate in rates for high and low performing ASCs.

IN SUMMARY

After fifty years of attempting to control the healthcare industry through regulation and rate setting, it is nothing short of stunning that, in March 2019, Med-Pac declared: "As we examine each of the payment systems, we also look for opportunities to develop policies that create incentives for providing high-quality care efficiently across providers and over time. Some of the current payment systems create strong incentives for increasing volume, and very few of these systems encourage providers to work together toward common goals."[177]

The report continued:

> Alternative payment models (e.g., the Next Generation accountable care organization model) are meant to stimulate delivery system reform toward more integrated and value-oriented health care systems and may address these issues. We will continue to contribute to their development and track their progress. In the near term, the Commission will continue to closely examine a broad set of indicators, make sure there is consistent pressure on providers to control their costs, and set a demanding standard for determining which sectors qualify for a payment update each year.[178]

Imagine what it is like for members of Congress and their staff to read, attempt to comprehend, and continually update the legislation to deal with the mess created by this regulated environment.

It is, in fact, mind boggling.[179]

MedPac puts out two reports annually, each one now containing approximately 500 pages of such data. And this is just from a Medicare overview perspective. There are similar reports to Congress by the legislative committee (MACPAC) on the Medicaid system, as well as others from the Government Accounting Office (GAO), auditors, and the agencies themselves. The cost of this monitoring and supposedly independent advice for the legislators is staggering in and of itself.

CHAPTER 8

Hospital System Consolidation

FOLLOWING THE MONEY

After a half-century of trying to manage our healthcare delivery system and its cost, one outcome is clear: Medicare policy is driving the current, dangerous industry consolidation by hospital systems.

Two factors are at the heart of it.

First is the ACA legislation, with its goals and demo projects, which dictate hospital control of service delivery. Even though, as we have seen, the demos have been far from successful, they have provided the opportunity for hospitals to jump on the band wagon and gain more power and control.

Second is the highly favorable reimbursement for the range of services currently being assembled under the hospital system umbrella.

Medicare represents about one-third of hospital revenues and 44 percent of all admissions. Furthermore, as we saw in Chapter 1, Medicare policy and rates have an enormous effect on the entire healthcare industry and are thus of "critical importance" in shaping industry direction. The industry responds and will continue to respond to what it foresees as the will and desire of the regulators. Nothing illustrates this more dramatically than the current wave of consolidation and service delivery control by hospital systems.

MERGER AND ACQUISITION ACTIVITY
SINCE THE ACA ENACTMENT

In a September 18, 2018 *Wall Street Journal* article, Anna Wilde Mathews reported that, in 2010, the year the Affordable Care Act passed, the annual number of hospital mergers shot up 40%. The upswing has not abated since then. Mathews also noted that hospitals have been snapping up other types of providers, including doctor practices, clinics, and outpatient surgery centers.[180]

In March 2013, Medpac reported, "Hospital industry consolidation has increased in recent years, indicating that hospital systems still see acquisitions of other hospitals as a good use of their capital. ... Both the number of deals and the number of hospitals involved in the 2011 deals represent a marked increase from 2009 and 2010. For the third consecutive year, most of these hospital deals involved regional hospital systems acquiring either smaller local hospital systems or small independent hospitals."[181] The March 2019 MedPac report noted: "in 2015, the number of hospital mergers increased 18 percent from the prior year and 70 percent from 2010 (Ellison 2016)."[182]

Tim Mullaney reported in 2018:

Transformative mergers and acquisitions took place in health care last year. ... In 2017, there [was] ... the highest level of activity in at least 17 years, according to a new report from Kaufman Hall. ... Hospitals and health systems are now looking to diversify their business lines, compelled by a broad range of objectives. These include building a stronger brand and presence, network infrastructure, risk-bearing capabilities, care continuum, and diversified operations, according to the report." The article stated that in 2017 the acquisitions tended to occur across regions rather than in the same market, and that such acquisitions result in greater market power for hospitals, in both the individual market and regional context, and in negotiating contracts with insurers, physicians, and drug and device manufacturers.[183]

Mathews's Sept. 18, 2018 *Wall Street Journal* article points out that "Dominant hospital systems use an array of secret contract terms to protect their turf and block efforts to curb health-care costs." They can "demand insurers include them in every plan and discourage use of less-expensive rivals." They also include clauses which allow them to "mask prices from consumers, limit audits of claims, add extra fees and block efforts to exclude health-care providers based on quality or cost." Just as disturbing was the fact that such "restrictive hospital-insurer contracts have helped prevent even big employers, including Walmart and Home Depot Inc., from moving forward with plans they were exploring to try to lower costs and improve quality for their workers." Mathews found dozens of such contracts with major hospital systems, which were "able to command advantageous terms because they have grown through years of deal-making, shifting the balance of power between hospitals and insurers." They found that hospitals can essentially set their price if they are a single or dominant system in a region. It also cited a study published in April in the Journal of Health Economics which found that doctors' prices increased on average by 14.1% after they became part of hospital systems.[184]

In March 2018, MedPac reported: "Regulators and researchers have noted concerns about increased consolidations and their effect on prices. ... Hospitals and physician groups have increasingly consolidated, in part to gain leverage over insurers in negotiating higher payment rates."[185] In March 2019, the commission stated that, as verified by many research reports, a "key driver" in the per capita spending growth on health care spending in the private sector between 2010 and 2016 was provider market power and further noted, "Increased consolidation has an inflationary effect on prices paid in the private sector. A recent study found that disparity in hospital prices within regions is the primary driver of variation in health care spending for the privately insured (Cooper et al., 2015). The study shows that hospitals that face few competitors have substantially higher prices."[186] This may be so, but far more important drivers have been the bundled payment and other demo projects created as a result of the ACA legislation, as we have seen. Below, we will address another principal driver: ill-conceived Medicare pricing policies.

As the Mergers and Acquisitions would indicate, financial position in the hospital industry is strong. In March 2019, MedPac noted:

Hospitals' access to capital for expansions and acquisitions is largely dependent on their total (all-payer) profitability. ... Operating margins (which exclude investment income) peaked in 2015 at 6.4 percent after a growth in insured patients. In 2017, total margins (which include investment income) were 7.1 percent, near an all-time high [7.2% in 2013; see p. .66]. Other measures of all-payer profitability are also strong. Cash flow—as measured by earnings before interest, taxes, depreciation, and amortization (EBITDA)—has remained steady and strong for the past eight years, between 10 percent and 11 percent. Financial ratings agencies consistently reported in 2018 that for-profit and nonprofit financial balance sheets (which include measures such as EBITDA, days cash on hand, and debt load) were at historically high levels for the industry (Barclays 2018, Fitch Ratings 2018, Moody's Investors Service 2018, S&P Global Ratings 2018).[187]

One of the major areas of acquisitions is physician practices. On June 2, 2018, Shelby Livingston, of *Modern Healthcare,* reported:

> Hospital systems are buying physician practices at an amazing rate, and can afford it in order to keep clients in their system at the higher rates that Medicare pays them. A Brookings Institute study found that 40% of hospital admissions are reported to come from hospital-owned physician practices. A study by the consulting firm Avalere Health and the Physicians Advocacy Institute, found that hospital systems acquired 5,000 independent practices that employed 14,000 physicians in the year between July 2015 and July 2016. This represented an 11% increase, on top of an 86% increase between 2012 and 2015. By July 2016, 42% of physicians were employed by hospitals, and the pace of consolidation only continues to advance. A 2018 Survey of America's Physicians found that only 31.4% of physicians identified as independent practice owners or partners.[188]

The "vanishing individual practitioner," was reporter Livingston's major concern in writing the *Modern Healthcare* article. Indeed, the direct purchase of physician practices by hospital systems has spurred other competitive shifts from solo and small practices to larger practices, as MedPac discussed in March 2019, citing an Irving Levin Associates study from 2016, which discussed a 47% jump in hospital related and independent transactions in 2014. MedPac also cited a 2015 Government Accountability Office (GAO) report, which found that, between 2007 and 2013, the number of physicians in "vertically consolidated" practices—hospital-acquired physician practices, physicians hired as salaried employees, or both—nearly doubled, and a 2016 Federal Trade Commission (FTC) report, which observed that all this activity has "significant implications for competition."[189]

Another area of acquisitions is skilled nursing facilities (SNFs). In March 2019, MedPac noted:

> Hospitals with SNFs can lower their inpatient lengths of stay by transferring patients to their SNF beds, thus making inpatient beds available to treat additional inpatient admissions. As a result, hospital based SNFs can contribute to the bottom-line financial performance of hospitals: Hospitals with SNFs had lower inpatient costs per case and higher inpatient Medicare margins than hospitals without SNFs.

In support of this statement about the importance of the ACA demo projects to the consolidation activity, the report goes on to observe, "The share of hospitals with financial links to SNFs has slowly increased as alternative payment models encourage hospitals to lower spending and improve clinical outcomes for services furnished in post-acute care. In 2015, 18 percent of hospitals had a financial link to a SNF, up from 11 percent in 2005 (Fowler et al. 2017)." The March 2018 Med-Pac report noted, "In the spring of 2017, CMS issued an advance notice of proposed rulemaking ... and sought comments on a redesign of the SNF PPS" in which "payments would shift from freestanding to hospital-based providers."[190]

It appears that Certified Home Health Agencies (HHAs) have always been a focus. The March 2019 MedPac report stated: "The Commission includes hospital HHAs in its calculation of acute care hospitals' Medicare margins because these agencies operate in the financial context of hospital operations. ... Hospital-based HHAs help their parent institutions financially if they can shorten inpatient stays, lowering stays in the most costly setting." On the same page, it discussed another benefit to hospital revenues, the fact that HHAs absorb "overhead costs allocated" to them from the parent hospital. This means that HHAs have higher costs than independent agencies.[191]

THE CONTRIBUTION OF ILL-CONCEIVED PRICING POLICIES

Outpatient services

MedPac (March 2019) stated that, from 2012 to 2017, Medicare spending for hospital outpatient services grew at an annual rate of 8.6 percent. Contributing to this strong growth rate were:

- Drug administration and the cost of drugs, especially for the treatment of cancer
- Emergency department visits and observation care
- Clinic visits, likely fueled by hospital acquisition of physician practices and hospital employment of physicians
- Complex surgical procedures, which often involve prosthetics or medical devices and that migrate from the inpatient setting[192]

Physician practices in hospital outpatient departments (HOPDs)

What would any intelligent person expect to happen when physicians in hospital settings are paid more than in private practice? Physicians will continue to sell their practices to hospitals, and the hospitals will use them to keep patients within their own system. That, in fact, is what is happening. From MedPac (March 2019):

> "Medicare makes both a fee schedule payment and a facility payment when a service is provided in an HOPD (the facility payment accounts for the cost of the service in an HOPD). However, the program makes only a fee schedule payment when a service is furnished in a freestanding office. For example, in 2018, the total payment for the most common E&M office/outpatient visit for an established patient when provided in an HOPD (other than certain off-campus HOPDs) was $166 ($52 for the fee schedule payment to the clinician plus $114 for the facility payment to the HOPD) compared with $74 (the nonfacility fee schedule payment) for this visit when provided in a freestanding office. … As of 2019, Medicare pays a comparable amount for E&M office/outpatient visits in freestanding physician offices and off-campus HOPDs (greater than 35 miles from the hospital); however, Medicare continues to pay a higher amount for these visits when provided in on-campus HOPDs."

> "The growth in service volume has contributed significantly to an increase in spending for fee schedule services …."[193]

In June of 2013, MedPac reported an "increased urgency to address payment variations across setting because many services have been migrating from physicians' offices to the usually higher paid OPD (outpatient department) setting as hospital employment of physicians has grown … resulting in higher program spending without significant changes in patient care."[194]

In March 2019, this discussion continued in MedPac, which reported:

Another large source of growth in spending on hospital outpatient services was a shift from (relatively lower cost) physician offices to (relatively higher cost) hospital outpatient departments (HOPDs). From 2012 to 2017, spending for, and the volume of, clinic visits and drug administration (especially for chemotherapy drugs) in the hospital outpatient setting rose substantially, while the volume of these services fell in freestanding physician offices.[195]

> "From 2011 to 2016, spending for and volume of clinic visits … rose substantially in the OPPS setting, while there was a decrease or only slight growth in volume of these services in freestanding physician offices. Over this period,

the volume of OPPS clinic visits increased by 43.8% (7.5 percent per year) … At the same time, the volume of office visits in freestanding offices rose by only 0.4 percent … The growth in volume in HOPDs over this period is reflected in increased spending on clinic visits, which rose by 76 percent (12.0 percent per year). This shift in care setting to HOPDs is important in that it increases Medicare program spending and beneficiary cost-sharing liability because Medicare payment rates for the same or similar services are generally higher in HOPDs than in freestanding offices. For example, we estimate that the Medicare program spent $1.8 billion more in 2016 than it would have if payment rates for evaluation and management (E&M) office visits in HOPDs were the same as freestanding office rates. Analogously, beneficiaries' cost sharing was $460 million more in 2016 than it would have been because of the higher rates paid in HOPDs."[196]

The March 2018 MedPac discussed the fact that "prior Commission reports have explored the relationship between inpatient, outpatient, and physician services and found that growth in outpatient services in part reflects hospitals purchasing freestanding physician practices and billing these services through the higher paying hospital outpatient prospective payment system." It went on to observe that, in 2012, it had recommended equalizing payment rates between physicians' office and hospital settings for 66 service categories to remove the financial incentive for hospitals to purchase physician practices.[197]

In March 2014, MedPac suggested equalizing the rates for even more service categories. The next year, the Bipartisan Budget Act of 2015 did require adjustment of the rates beginning in 2017—but only for "certain services" provided in "off-campus" clinics. The outcome of this legislative requirement was reported in the March 2019 MedPac, which found that hospitals simply switched to providing these services on their main campuses so that they could bill at the highest rates. MedPac also reported its finding that the market shift away from independent practice was clearly a "large source of growth in spending on hospital outpatient services," with clinic visits and volume rising 34%.[198]

Drugs
The 2019 March MedPAC found that the "largest source of OPPS spending growth has been Part B drugs." Between 2012 and 2017, Part B drug costs increased 99%, with 79% of the increase due to cancer treating drugs, including chemotherapy administration, which rose 45%. From 2016 to 2017, drug spending on off-campus Part B drugs grew 25.5% and accounted for nearly 29 percent

of the growth in total drug spending in hospital:

> The growth in combined program spending and cost sharing for drugs has accelerated in recent years (2016 to 2017), increasing 18.2 percent. … Drugs are profitable overall in the outpatient setting because hospitals' revenues exceed their costs for drugs, largely driven by the substantial margins for drugs obtained through the 340B Drug Pricing Program, a federal program that requires drug manufacturers to provide outpatient drugs to certain hospitals at significantly reduced prices.[199]

Emergency Departments (ED) and Urgent Care Centers (UCC)

The June 2019 MedPAC report stated:

> "Medicare beneficiaries have rapidly increased their use of UCCs, but hospital EDs remain a common setting for nonurgent care, which we define as care related to any physician claim on which the principal diagnosis code includes one of seven conditions: bronchitis, urinary tract infection, upper respiratory infection, sprain, contusion, back pain, or arthritis."

> "When a hospital ED treats a nonurgent condition, the Medicare program and beneficiaries spend between 3 and 20 times more per episode than when a UCC treats the same condition."

> "We estimate that about one-third of ED claims involving nonurgent care (or 2 percent of Medicare physician ED claims) could be appropriately treated in a UCC or other lower cost, non-ED setting."

> "Under the hospital outpatient prospective payment system (OPPS), hospitals code each ED visit into one of five levels of intensity, with Level 1 as the least resource intensive with the lowest payment rate and Level 5 as the most resource intensive with the highest payment rate. In 2005, ED visits across these five levels reflected an approximately normal distribution, with Level 3 as the most frequently coded level and Levels 1 and 5 as the least frequently coded. However, in recent years, coding of ED visits has steadily shifted to higher levels. In 2017, Level 4 was the most frequently coded level and Level 5 was the second most frequently coded. In 2017, hospitals coded 66 percent of ED visits as Level 4 or Level 5, up from 37 percent in 2005. Reportedly, coding of ED visits has shifted from lower levels to higher levels for patients covered by private insurance as well."[200]

> "The high concentration of ED visits coded as Level 5 suggests hospitals are potentially coding patients in response to payment incentives and Medicare is paying more than necessary for many patients who present in the ED setting."

"Medicare could change the system of ED codes to improve its payment accuracy. [Since (p. 386) there are no national guidelines for hospitals to refer to when coding ED visits,] Medicare could begin by developing a system of ED codes that are based on national coding guidelines and that reflect the resources hospitals use to treat ED patients."[201]

"The Current Procedural Terminology (CPT) codes that hospitals use to code ED visits reflect the work and resources of physicians, not hospitals. CMS has responded to this lack of CPT codes for hospitals by directing hospitals to develop their own internal guidelines for coding ED visits. ... We do not know much about the coding guidelines hospitals use, but the definitions are likely to vary. The lack of national guidelines for hospitals makes identifying differences in hospital resource use problematic and makes auditing hospital coding more difficult."[202]

"Medicare regulates UCCs by designating them as equivalent to physician offices. An encounter by a Medicare beneficiary at a UCC triggers one of two payment scenarios, depending on the facility's hospital affiliation: If an encounter is at an independent UCC (not affiliated with a hospital), it generates only a PFS claim. The UCC receives the same higher nonfacility-based PFS payment rate as physician offices and retail clinics. UCCs use 1 of 10 evaluation and management (E&M) codes to characterize each visit and bill separately for ancillary services. These facilities cannot bill Medicare for one of the five ED CPT codes.

"If the encounter is at a UCC that is a provider-based department of a hospital, it generates both a PFS claim and an OPPS claim. The PFS claim for the clinician services includes 1 of the 10 E&M codes and is paid using the facility-based PFS payment rates, which are lower than the nonfacility rates. Under the PFS, some ancillary services are also separately paid. The OPPS claim for the facility services uses a single code for a hospital outpatient clinic visit.

"Medicare payment rates are generally higher for comparable patients when they are treated in a hospital ED, relative to a UCC. Under a hypothetical example of the most common ED level—a Level 4 ED visit—the 2019 Medicare payment rate for a hospital ED open 24/7 is $480, combining the PFS payment of $120 and the OPPS payment of $360 (not including other ancillary services) (Figure 11-1). By contrast, if the same patient were treated in an independent UCC, the UCC would receive a nonfacility-based PFS payment of $167. Because beneficiaries in all of these settings are responsible for 20 percent cost sharing, their liability differs greatly depending on where the service is provided."[203]

In 2017, 8 of the 20 most common conditions treated at UCCs were also among the 20 most common conditions treated at hospital EDs: urinary tract infections, cough, hypertension, back pain, pneumonia, dizziness, chest pain, and shortness of breath. Compared with EDs, UCCs tend to serve a larger share of beneficiaries who are established patients (as opposed to new patients).

The June 2018 MedPac report addressed the subject of "off-campus" emergency departments (OCEDs). These are hospital-owned units, which can get the same rate as the on-campus ED if it is less than 35 miles from the hospital and has 24-hour access. If it does not have 24-hour access, the rate is discounted 30%. However, even the discounted rate is double what the urgent care center or physician's office down the street would get. With this competitive advantage, "the number of OCEDs has increased rapidly in recent years, particularly in areas with high household incomes." Thus, services are migrating from physician offices to off-campus EDs. MedPac believed that, since these facilities don't take trauma and other cases on-campus EDs accept, rates should be lowered 30%. Doing this would save $50 million to $250 million annually.[204]

Some micro hospitals (fewer than ten beds) focus on ED services. They typically offer a limited range of services but can bill Medicare at the OPPS rates, which are "substantially more" than PFS rates. This led MedPac to conclude that they also might be getting overpaid for the ED and outpatient services they perform.[205]

Technology Pass-throughs

In March 2002, MedPac reported:

> The pass-through system makes additional payments to hospitals for certain new technology items based on hospitals' reported costs and manufacturers' prices. The current mechanism creates incentives to manufacturers and hospitals to raise their prices and charges, and will eventually result in incorrect relative payments among all outpatient services ... These flaws in the payment system have been highlighted because administrative and legislative actions dramatically increased the number of items entering the pass-through pool.[206]

Observation Care and Emergency Department usage

The March 2018 MedPac reported that, along with other outpatient services, spending "rose substantially for observation care and emergency department (ED) visits. ... From 2011 to 2016, OPPS (Outpatient Prospective Payment

System) spending for observation care increased by 349 percent (35.0 percent per year). ... In this same period, OPPS spending for ED visits increased by 76 percent (11.9 percent per year). It is not clear what caused this increase in observation stays and ED visits, but the increase may be due, in part, to reactions to denials for certain short inpatient stays and the introduction in fiscal year 2014 of a two-midnight rule for inpatient stays (Medicare Payment Advisory Commission 2015a)." It went on to state that, in the 2015 to 2016 timeframe, there was also a 76% rate increase due to a CMS decision to redefine observation care. The idea behind the decision was "to combine all services [otherwise] recorded on an outpatient claim into a single payment." This was combined with a "slightly stronger criteria that needed to be met ... for the observation care to be paid." Although these changes resulted in a decrease of 5% in the volume of cases, the net result was an "approximately 75 percent increase in payments for observation care." [207]

The March 2019 MedPac report continued to report increases, noting that OPPS spending "has increased substantially for observation care. From 2012 to 2017, OPPS spending for observation care rose 263 percent, attributable to higher volume, updates to OPPS payment rates, and a substantial increase in the ancillary items included in the packaged payment rate for observation care in 2016." Likewise, "OPPS spending for emergency department (ED) visits ... increased, rising by 72 percent from 2012 to 2017."

> Similar to observation care, a number of factors contributed to the increase in spending on ED visits, including increased volume, updates to the ED payment rates, increased packaging of ancillary items into the ED payment rates, and a shift of ED visits coded at lower acuity levels to higher acuity levels. ... Finally, we have found that a shift in the coding of ED visits from low-acuity levels (which have lower payment rates) to higher acuity levels (which have higher payment rates) increased ED spending by 20.3 percent from 2012 to 2017. [208]

Surgical services in Hospital Outpatient Departments (HOPDs)

In March 2018, MedPac reported:

> The hospital outpatient setting has had higher growth in program spending than any other sector in Medicare. From 2011 through 2016, combined program spending and beneficiary cost sharing on services covered under the OPPS increased by 51 percent, from $39.8 billion to $60.0 billion, an average of 8.6 percent per year." The 2018 "Medicare payment rates are 92 percent higher in hospital outpatient departments (under a separate hospital outpatient prospective payment system (OPPS) than in ASCs [209]

The March 2018 report continued:

A reason for the higher growth of surgical services in HOPDs relative to ASCs [Ambulatory Surgery Centers] over the 2011 through 2016 period may be that Medicare payment rates have become much higher in HOPDs than in ASCs, which might make it less financially attractive to provide surgical services for Medicare patients in ASCs ... physicians continue to move away from working in private practices toward working for hospitals or medical groups (Merritt Hawkins 2014, Physicians Advocacy Institute 2016). Physicians working for hospitals may be more inclined to perform procedures at the hospitals that employ them than at freestanding ASCs. ... [however] Maintaining beneficiaries' access to ASCs is beneficial because services provided in this setting are less costly to Medicare and beneficiaries than services delivered in HOPDs. ... This issue is pertinent ... because among even the most frequently provided services in ASCs, a substantial volume is provided in HOPDs.[210]

Because Medicare's payment systems were developed independently and have had different update trajectories, payments for similar services can vary widely. For example, under the current payment systems, ... the same physician could see the same patient and provide the same service, but depending on whether the service is provided in an outpatient clinic or in a physician's office, Medicare's payment and the beneficiary's coinsurance can differ by 80 percent or more.[211]

•

The sobering lesson of the consolidation in the American healthcare industry, headlong in tempo and unprecedented in magnitude, is that fifty years of heedlessly arrogant healthcare regulation has distorted the marketplace in ways beyond what any prior federal regulatory regime ever contemplated. In the United States, government regulation of the free market has its origins in the early twentieth-century Progressive era of Teddy Roosevelt. Back then, it was chiefly about "trust busting," breaking up the monopolies—beginning with the petroleum industry—that menaced the free market to the detriment of consumers. During the last half-century, however, the frenzied efforts to socialize healthcare, to impose upon the industry a centrally regulated command economy, has grotesquely distorted even the best intentions of Progressivism. With this, the taxpayer and the consumer—who is also the patient, seeking cost-effective, state-of-the-art healthcare—is left to struggle with payment of an unjust and unjustifiable bill.

The Elusive "Value-Based Care"

Fifty years of bureaucratic micromanagement, thousands of demo projects, and hundreds of billions of dollars have failed to produce the policy goal of "value-based care." The question for Congress: Why continue down this road? It is time for a total change in direction.

In one of the greatest understatements of our time, MedPac stated in its March 2019 report: "Certain structural features of the Medicare program pose challenges for targeting inefficient spending." This was followed by another understatement, only slightly less stupendous: "However, the Commission has made multiple recommendations to the Congress and the Secretary that have the potential to improve the quality of care and move the Medicare program toward paying for value."[212]

MedPac has been making recommendations to Congress and CMS for twenty years. The last three chapters of this book have illustrated how little effect these recommendations have had either in identifying quality or identifying the proper price for efficient delivery of service. Consider this, from March 2019—and understand that its context has been reiterated in every March MedPac report since March 2012. In fact, the statements in italics have been reproduced, word for word, every year:

A core principle guiding the Commission is that Medicare should pay the same amount for the same service, even when it is provided in different settings. Putting this principle into practice requires that the definition of services in the settings and the characteristics of the patients be sufficiently similar. Where these conditions are not met, offsetting adjustments would have to be made to ensure comparability. *Because Medicare's payment systems were developed independently and have had different update trajectories, payments for similar services can vary widely. Such differences create opportunities for Medicare and beneficiary savings if payment is set at the level applicable to the lowest priced setting in which the service can be safely performed.* For example, under the current payment systems, a beneficiary can receive the same physician visit service in a hospital outpatient clinic or in a physician's office. In fact, the same physician could see the same patient and provide the same service, but depending on whether the service is provided in an outpatient clinic or in a physician's office, Medicare's payment and the beneficiary's coinsurance can differ by 80 percent or more.

This service is comparable across the two settings. Our recommendation sets payment rates for E&M office visits both in the outpatient department and physician office sectors equal to those in the physician fee schedule, lowering both program spending and beneficiary liability (Medicare Payment Advisory Commission 2012). In 2014, we extended that principle to additional services for which payment rates in the outpatient PPS should be lowered to better match payment rates in the physician office setting (Medicare Payment Advisory Commission 2014). In the Bipartisan Budget Act of 2015, the Congress made payment for outpatient departments for the same services equal to the physician fee schedule rates for those services at any new outpatient off-campus clinic beginning in 2018. We also recommended consistent payment between acute care hospitals and long-term care hospitals for certain categories of patients (Medicare Payment Advisory Commission 2014). In 2016, we recommended elements of a unified PAC PPS that would make payments based on a patient's needs and characteristics, generally irrespective of the PAC entity that provided their care (Medicare Payment Advisory Commission 2016). *The Commission will continue to study other services that are provided in multiple sites of care to find additional services for which the principle of the same payment for the same service can be applied.*

The Medicare Prescription Drug, Improvement, and Modernization Act of 2003 requires the Commission to consider the budgetary consequences of our recommendations. Therefore, this report documents how spending for each recommendation would compare with expected spending under current law.

It is essential to look at payment adequacy not only within the context of individual payment systems but also in terms of Medicare as a whole. *The Commission is concerned by any increase in Medicare spending per beneficiary without a commensurate increase in value such as higher quality of care or improved health status.* Growth in spending per beneficiary, combined with the aging of the baby boomers, will result in the Medicare program absorbing increasing shares of the gross domestic product and federal spending. Medicare's rising costs are projected to exhaust the Hospital Insurance Trust Fund (which funds Medicare Part A) and significantly burden taxpayers. Ensuring that the recent moderate growth trends in Medicare spending per beneficiary continue will require vigilance. *The financial future of Medicare prompts us to look at payment policy and ask what can be done to develop, implement, and refine payment systems to reward quality and efficient use of resources while improving payment equity.*

In many past reports, the Commission has stated that Medicare should institute policies that improve the program's value to beneficiaries and taxpayers. CMS is beginning to take such steps, and we discuss them in the sector-specific chapters that follow. Ultimately, increasing Medicare's value to beneficiaries and taxpayers requires knowledge about the costs and health outcomes of services. Until more information about the comparative effectiveness of new and existing health care treatments and technologies is available, patients, providers, and the program will have difficulty determining what constitutes high-quality care and effective use of resources.

As we examine each of the payment systems, we also look for opportunities to develop policies that create incentives for providing high-quality care efficiently across providers and over time. Some of the current payment systems create strong incentives for increasing volume, and very few of these systems encourage providers to work together toward common goals. Alternative payment models (e.g., the Next Generation accountable care organization model) are meant to stimulate delivery system reform toward more integrated and value-oriented health care systems and may address these issues.

In the near term, the Commission will continue to closely examine a broad set of indicators, make sure there is consistent pressure on providers to control their costs, and set a demanding standard for determining which sectors qualify for a payment update each year. In the longer term, pressure on providers may cause them to increase their participation in alternative payment models. We will continue to contribute to the development of those models and to increase their efficacy.[213]

As we have seen, the quest for value-based care and the recommendations to achieve it were ongoing long before 2012, have continued through 2019, and unless the course is changed, will continue far into the future. Note the many recommendations constantly restated by MedPac. Note the inability to demonstrate any implementation or success, as we have seen throughout this book. And finally, note that variations on the same demonstration models continue even as the goalpost has been carefully and quietly moved—with authorization, wittingly or not, of Congress. The aim is now "delivery system reform," as we discussed in Chapter 6, which has led to the industry consolidation covered in Chapter 8. This aim continues despite the concerns of regulators and researchers cited in the March 2019 report about consolidation and its effect on pricing and about the lack of success with the demo projects.[214]

The March 2012 MedPac report shows that the commission has entertained the notion that industry consolidation could "make it easier for Medicare reforms to diffuse across markets" and could "present an opportunity to control overall costs under Medicare by controlling the volume of services and by providing greater care coordination."[215] This idea has been disproved by failed demo projects and by the simple fact that prices continue to skyrocket with the market consolidation that has taken place.

And in 2019, MedPac was still making serious admissions:

- "The Medicare program is a complex and fragmented system, consisting of multiple paths to entitlement; multiple types of coverage (Part A, Part B, Part C (Medicare Advantage), and Part D); multiple payment systems; and different rules for each setting. The Medicare program must set prices for thousands of discrete services at different levels of aggregation (e.g., inpatient hospital payments are paid based on the stay, while physician payments are based on the service) and in different labor markets across the country. The Medicare program statute and rulemaking include a substantial number of exceptions, adjustments, and modifications to its general policies. Several of Medicare's structural features (and some shared across the health care system) complicate efforts to achieve spending efficiencies."

- "The program sets payment rates each year for at least nine health care settings or provider types: acute care hospitals, physician and other health professional services, home health agencies, skilled nursing facilities, long-term care facilities, hospice, inpatient rehabilitation facilities, ambulatory surgical centers, and end-stage renal disease dialysis facilities. In addition to the yearly rule-making process involved in setting these rates, administrators oversee other parts of the program that operate on fee schedules (ambulances, outpatient lab facilities) or on cost-based payment (rural health centers, critical access hospitals). Payment rates for Part C (Medicare Advantage) are set using administrative pricing based on a competitive process, and Part D payments (prescription drugs) are generally set by market rates. The fragmented payment system across multiple health care settings reduces incentives to provide patient-centered, coordinated care."

- "In the process of setting rates for thousands of services, certain services are undervalued relative to others, providing incorrect incentives for their use. For example, the Commission has raised concerns that the Medicare fee schedule overpays for services provided by clinicians in procedural specialties and underpays for services provided by clinicians in primary care specialties (Medicare Payment Advisory Commission 2011a). This imbalance results in significantly higher income for clinicians in procedural specialties relative to those in primary care specialties, contributing to a corresponding imbalance in clinician supply."

- "The Congress has recognized the need for CMS to pursue value-based purchasing policies. For example, the Improving Medicare Post-Acute Care Transformation Act of 2014 required post-acute care providers to report standardized performance data and linked these measures to payment. Earlier, in 2010, the PPACA emphasized tying payment to quality in the Medicare program (e.g., by allowing accountable care organizations that meet quality thresholds to share in cost savings and by reducing payments to hospitals with excessive readmissions and hospital-acquired conditions). The PPACA also included new CMS authorities through the establishment of an innovation center to test different payment structures and methodologies; the intention is to reduce program expenditures while maintaining or improving quality of care, which, if successful, could be extended across Medicare."[216]

In other words, MedPac has admitted that nothing has worked.

In March 2019, MedPac stated that, from 1975 to 2009, total health care spending and Medicare spending grew robustly, annually averaging 9.0 percent and 10.6 percent, respectively. Although from 2009 to 2013 the rate of increase slowed to 3.7 percent and 4.3 percent, respectively, it increased to 5.5 and 4.9 percent respectively from 2013 to 2015 and has been rising much faster than the rate of inflation since then.[217]

The fact is that the entire Medicare program was ill-conceived from the beginning and has undergone many ill-conceived modifications (like the mandated PPS system) over the last 50 years. It is simply foolish, given the complexity of the marketplace and the lack of success in defining care delivery systems, quality, and setting pricing for the services produced, that Congress, MedPac, and CMS would move on to attempting delivery system reform. Unfortunately, under the ACA legislation of 2010, Congress has authorized precisely this, and it has given a virtually free hand to the Secretary to carry out its hopeless decision.

Why does Congress waste its time with innumerable bills aimed at controlling the system and attempting to stem runaway costs? Why create and keep expanding the bureaucracy and budget to continue the doomed effort to achieve these impossible goals?

As this 50-year history demonstrates, we cannot design, manipulate, or control 20% of our economy from a bureaucratic armchair and expect to get the best product at the best price. To attain the goal of true reform, we must change our orientation.

It is time to leave benefit administration up to the bureaucrats but put operations in the hands of professionals in a competitive marketplace. The professionals are confident enough of their expertise to enter a marketplace and risk their investment to win consumers with innovative, high quality services and competitive prices. The marketplace capable of enticing such professionals to participate must offer freedom to enter, and it must encourage entrepreneurship, innovation, and competition. Such a marketplace will be alive and vibrant, instantly adjusting to consumer demands and technological advances. It will be professionally exciting and rewarding.

As Robert Helms wrote in his March 1, 1999 article for AEI:

> After 34 years of experience, we now know that the basic design of Medicare was fundamentally flawed. The government is a poor substitute for the discipline of the marketplace. Even when the creation of a government program creates great monopoly power in the purchase of services, government does not have the ability to control the cost of the program while keeping consumers satisfied. Market-based approaches to reform have the advantage of keeping consumers' and producers' incentives in line and continually reminding everyone, even vote-seeking politicians, that there are limits on what even the wealthiest nation in the world can spend on medical care.[218]

"Market-based approaches" are the sum and substance of the simple solution hidden by the aura of "complexity" created by the bureaucrats and the providers in a system that has both entrenched and enshrined their positions. The truth? Healthcare is not different from any other industry. It has simply been stymied by regulation and regulators. The healthcare marketplace is not free to enter but is restricted by certificate of need (CON) allotments and other regulatory provisions. Likewise, smothered by regulation and prodded into monopolistic consolidation, the market is not competitive. It is not vibrant. It does not adjust to consumer needs or technological advancements the way it should. Instead, it is hobbled by a combination of entrenched positions, absence of competitive spirit, and mountains of regulations controlling operations and stifling innovation. Instead, it relies on centrally conceived ideas, and demo projects needing years and billions of dollars to bring to conclusion. If these projects are not stillborn, irrelevant or obsolete by the time they are initiated, they surely meet this fate by the time they are concluded. They are costly projects whose only value lay in providing endless jobs for central planners and providers who would not otherwise survive. Instead of allowing competition to eliminate operators that don't meet the expectations of the marketplace, the bureaucrats arbitrarily establish and enforce their own quality standards, which protect the poorest performers.

When everything is codified down to how often, and in what form, a social worker must report to the administration, the industry becomes stagnant. When the regulations dictate the classifications of facilities and what they can or cannot do, the industry becomes stagnant. When providers have no fear of market-disrupting competition, the industry becomes both complacent and stagnant. When operators cannot try their own ideas without encountering staggering regulatory hurdles and without waiting years for regulatory changes, the industry becomes stagnant. When operations are run by the book, with pre-established rates and a paralyzing fear of being seen as a market disrupter, the industry becomes stagnant.

When the healthcare industry is stagnant, the consumer suffers.

For 50 years we have had a marketplace designed and controlled by those without industry expertise. And now we have reached a crossroads. The ACA has quietly, yet at staggering cost, continued to take us down the bureaucratic and non-professional pathway. It is now leading the industry to a level of consolidation that will be very difficult to reverse.

The time to act to change course is upon us. We soon will have an industry run by bureaucrats, hospital systems, and insurance companies (if these even continue to exist). Whatever competition and innovation remain today will be gone tomorrow and almost impossible to replace.

It is time to face facts. No government official or agency has the wherewithal to even imagine that they possess the infinite wisdom or even the basic expertise to design, control, or anticipate how an entire segment of the economy should operate. Furthermore, Congress should not legislate that an agency be responsible for such a task. Likewise, a government agency purchasing goods and services without any assurance that those services are of value or that the prices being paid are reasonable should cease and desist from its current operations. And last, it must be realized that no one has any idea how efficiently and effectively goods and services can be delivered without letting barriers to entry fall, and competition to flourish.

A fundamental change in the industry structure must be made immediately. We must move to eliminate the laws and regulations at the state and federal levels hindering free market activity. We must allow the marketplace to establish the most efficient mechanisms of care delivery and at what price care can be delivered. The arbitrary classifications of providers and what services they are permitted to deliver needs to end. It is time for innovative thinking. If the shackles are released in this marketplace, entrepreneurship and competition will be revived, tremendous innovations in care delivery and quality will be unleashed, and prices will drop at least 40%, virtually overnight. Information will flow, transparency will cease to be a scarce commodity, and consumer choice will reign.

The bonus will be untold billions of taxpayer dollars saved per year as the cost of needless bureaucratic management and regulation disappears.

Had Congress used "reasonable charges" as a basis for reimbursement of in-patient facilities and not attempted to design the whole system, competition among providers would have brought charges down to the point Congress itself was looking for—namely, reasonable cost plus a reasonable return on equity. Only the efficient providers would have survived, and quality levels and innovation in service delivery would have far outstripped what we see today. Furthermore, the subsidization of Medicaid and Medicare by private rates would have ended, and Medicaid patients would have equal access to high-quality providers.

The ACA legislation and the present push by CMS to reform the delivery of care is in conflict with Section 1801 of the Social Security Act (SSA), which states: "Nothing in this title shall be construed to authorize any Federal officer or employee to exercise any supervision or control over the practice of medicine or the manner in which medical services are provided."

THE SELF-INSURED LEAD THE WAY

Look at what is happening in the market at the current time. Walmart and the other large self-insured employers are doing their best to push value-based care for their employees by using sole-source contracting with various hospitals and physicians that have demonstrated expertise and efficiency in certain procedures and diseases. They are tired of insurers establishing pricing based on some sort of alignment with Medicare prices, and they are not waiting for government quality-of-care studies or using government provider ratings. Unless those providers who were left out in this contracting have been rendered totally unresponsive, paralyzed by the current regulated and protected environment, the success of large self-insured programs must stir some concern over lost business. It must stimulate at least the contemplation of a necessary competitive response, even if the business-loss exposure is currently envisioned as limited.

It is true, we should note, that sole-source contracting by large employers or co-ops of employers has been tried before, and it has ultimately failed. Perhaps the current attempts to find value-based care will not meet the same doom, but swimming against the tide of government regulation, related politics, demo projects, limited competition, and protected positions within the industry is not easy. Anna Wilde Mathews and Joseph Walker commented on this hard and well-traveled road "to change a complex and entrenched industry" in their February 1, 2018 article in the *Wall Street Journal* as they covered the planned venture by Amazon, Berkshire Hathaway and JPMorgan Chase to overhaul their workers' health care. They quoted Lonny Reisman, a former executive at Aetna Inc., who helped create an employer coalition in the 1990s that crafted deals with health-maintenance organizations. Mr. Reisman asked and answered: Do employer groups "have enough clout to actually change the nature of health-care delivery and pricing?"

"I don't think they've been very successful," he replied.[219]

However, while the state and federal governments are buried in demo projects projected to stretch well over a decade in their attempts to tease out quality and devise novel methods of delivering and paying for care, Walmart and the other large employers are forging ahead to find providers not only to deliver the highest quality and most efficient services currently available, but who have the internal processes necessary to constantly improve and innovate so that they will continue to deliver the best services into the future. If there were a free market, these competitive forces would swiftly impact product offerings and pricing throughout the industry. A glimpse of this potential was seen on January 30, 2018 when, as noted in the above- mentioned WSJ article, health care stocks were shaken by a mere news release of the planned venture by these large employers.

Tremors are also being created as other healthcare ventures, working within the current regulatory confines, attempt to deliver value-based solutions for the consumer. At the retail level, Walmart is making a foray into "partnering with local providers to deliver high-quality care" by opening health clinics in its stores wherever regulatory provisions allow, and as discussed in the last chapter, despite the comparatively lower reimbursement it will receive. Marcus Osborne, the VP of Walmart's health and wellness program, stated that Walmart is "committed to making healthcare more affordable (offering "prices at about 30 to 50 percent less") and accessible for customers in the communities Walmart serves without sacrificing quality." Osborne stated that Walmart is moving forward to "ensure" its own "value-based model." It is also putting its own capital at risk to pursue this venture and moving very rapidly to test and perfect the concept.[220]

As the Healthline article reported, Walmart is not alone trying to deliver better healthcare alternatives. It has competitors, all of which are trying to drive their own value-based propositions. Retail competitors including Target, Walgreens, CVS, and Rite Aid have all jumped in with different service offerings, and partnerships (such as with physician groups, labs, insurers and tech companies). All of them are putting their own capital at stake to develop their own value-based propositions for the customer, with no guarantee of success. The customer will be the ultimate judge. Pricing will have to be very competitive, and the consumer will be the winner. On February 24, 2020, Anna Wilde Mathews had an article in the *Wall Street Journal,* discussing how CVS is eliminating co-payments for Aetna members who use its clinics. She also noted a new insurance plan that Blue Cross & Blue Shield of Texas is offering that includes free primary care at clinics it recently opened with a partner. That plan is priced 12-18% below other products it offers, for it expects to reduce the use of emergency rooms and improve on usage of preventative care techniques. She stated that a Florida Blue's plan is doing likewise, and trying to achieve the same sort of results by driving patients to specialists and other healthcare providers that deliver the best outcomes. All of these ventures are doing the best they can under the present regulatory structure to bring value to the client, which in this case means zero out-of-pocket costs wherever possible, and lower plan premiums.[221]

THE OPPORTUNITIES FOR IMPROVEMENT
AND SAVINGS ARE ENDLESS

The projects discussed above can only provide a brief glimpse of the potential that could be unleashed if the marketplace was allowed to function properly. Free up the system and the opportunities are endless. The value equation would never stop improving.

Only one thing is necessary to bring us to this new level of sanity in health-care. It is a change in political and cultural orientation that will enable the collective decision to abandon a regulated environment and allow a free marketplace to deliver the desired program benefits at the best price.

No longer will we have to put up with providers that don't know their costs and cannot deliver the consumer desired value proposition. No longer will we be obliged to tolerate management of the system by government officials who have no comprehension of the dynamics of the industry, and what the consumer considers quality or value. No longer will we have to put up with a healthcare system that is decades behind in orientation.

No longer will Congress have to waste so much of its time hawking legislation governing subject matter it does not and cannot be expected to understand.

THE GREAT EXCEPTION

Consider this. One demo program is an exception to the long record of failure. Just one has shown tremendous success. It is competitive bidding.

The Durable Medical Equipment and Supplies (DMEPOS) Program

The June 2018 MedPac report stated that, due to rate setting based on supplier charges and adjusting payment rates for inflation over time, many DMEPOS products had become "substantially overpriced."[222]

The Balanced Budget Act of 1997 instructed the Secretary of HHS to conduct a competitive bidding demonstration (CBP) for durable medical equipment and supplies (DMEPOS). An initial demonstration carried out in Florida and Texas between 1999 and 2002 proved very successful, reducing Medicare expenditures by 19%. After this triumph, the Medicare Prescription Drug, Improvement, and Modernization Act of 2003 required another competitive bidding demonstration, this time to be held in ten of the nation's largest metropolitan areas, with a focus on the highest-cost and highest-volume items. Eight years later, in 2011, "Round 1" began in nine areas and had three competitions. "Round 2" began in 2013 in 90 metropolitan areas and had two competitions. There was also a special National Mail-Order Program for diabetes testing supplies. In 2016, CMS was using the pricing information gained through the competitions to adjust payment rates in other areas of the country not covered by the competitions. As of 2018, two competitions were still active.

The results of the CBP have been nothing short of phenomenal, a bright light in an otherwise dismal tunnel of a half-century of failed programs. In June 2018, MepPAC reported: "The CBP has successfully driven down the cost of DMEPOS products for the Medicare program and beneficiaries. Compared with payment rates in the year before the CBP, Medicare's payment rates for some of the highest expenditure DMEPOS products have fallen by an average of roughly 50 percent. ... At the same time, Medicare expenditures for DMEPOS products excluded from the CBP have continued to grow."[223] The 2018 report went on:

- "By 2015, nearly half of all Medicare expenditures on DMEPOS products were for products excluded from the CBP. Medicare pays for these products either using a fee schedule that is largely based on supplier charges from 1986 to 1987 (updated for inflation) and undiscounted list prices. Medicare's payment rates for the top 10 non-CBP DMEPOS products in 2015 were a third higher, on average, than private-payer rates for comparable products. Many non-CBP DMEPOS products continue to generate high rates of improper payments and utilization growth, and to exhibit patterns of potential fraud and abuse. To address these issues, additional products that are not currently competitively bid could be moved into the CBP."

- "Medicare expenditures on DMEPOS products included in the CBP have decreased considerably over time. From 2010 to 2015, Medicare expenditures for products included in the CBP fell from $7.5 billion to $4.4 billion, a decrease of 42 percent. Expenditures for certain types of products in the CBP declined even faster. For example, between 2010 and 2015, Medicare expenditures on diabetes testing supplies (e.g., blood glucose test strips) fell from $1.6 billion to $0.3 billion, a decrease of 79 percent (Table 6-1, p. 138)."

- "Over the same time period, Medicare expenditures on DMEPOS products not included in the CBP continued to increase. Between 2010 and 2015, expenditures for these products grew from $3.3 billion to $4.0 billion, a total increase of 23 percent. Because of the decrease in spending on CBP products and the increase in spending on non-CBP products, the share of total Medicare DMEPOS spending attributable to non-CBP products has increased rapidly. In 2010, non-CBP products represented about 30 percent of Medicare DMEPOS spending; by 2015, non-CBP products accounted for nearly half (48 percent) of all spending."

- "For DMEPOS products, the CBP has effectively used market competition to reduce payment rates and limit fraud and abuse for over seven years." [224]

MedPac finally had a highly successful demo project to report, but it hardly gets honorable mention, and the topic has not been raised again since this report. The Commission concludes the chapter simply stating that Medicare could improve by adding additional products to the competitive bidding program. It is astonishing that MedPac did not recommend that the demo be expanded and deployed nationwide, or request that Congress authorize a similar demo aimed at delivery of services. [225]

In its March 2009 report, MedPac stated that "The Commission strongly promotes the policy principle that Medicare's payment systems should encourage efficiency in the provision of Medicare services. Competitive markets demand continual efficiency improvements from the workers and firms who pay the taxes used to finance Medicare." Yet, instead of contemplating the use of a competitive marketplace to reach its goal, MedPac recommended the continued use of administered pricing to "exert" financial pressure to duplicate what the competitive market could accomplish, and endless "adjustments" to the formulas "to encourage providers to produce a unit of service as efficiently as possible while maintaining quality." That is what MedPac continues to recommend, and the adjustments to the formulas continue to fail.[226]

The fact is that MedPac is not about to recommend putting the administrative bureaucracy out of business even though it has completely failed in its attempt to duplicate the results that could achieved in a competitive marketplace. It is up to Congress to act on its own and correct the legislative failures that it has continued to follow for the last 50 years. The time to act is now.

Glossary

ACA: Affordable Care Act

ASC: Ambulatory surgery center

CBO: Congressional Budget Office

CBP: Competitive Bidding Program

CMI: Center for Medicare and Medicaid Innovation

CMS: Department within the Department of Health and Human Services (HHS)

CON: Certificate of Need; issued by states to permit the establishment of health-care facilities

CPI: Consumer Price Index

DMEPOS: Durable medical equipment, prosthetics, orthotics, and supplies

DRG: Diagnosis Related Grouping; used for establishing payment rates for similar conditions

ED: Hospital emergency department

FFS: Medicare direct fee for service as opposed to being paid by a Medicare Advantage insurance plan

GAO: Government Accounting Office

GDP: U. S. Gross Domestic Product

HCPCS: Healthcare Common Procedure Coding System

HHA: Home Health Agency

HOPD: Hospital outpatient department

IRF: Inpatient rehabilitation facility

LTCH: Long term care hospital

MA: Medicare Advantage

Medicaid: Joint federal and state program under SSA Title XIX covering care for low-income individuals

Medicare SSA Title XVIII: Federal Health Insurance program for those over age 65

Medicare Part A: An entitlement program covering hospital and post-acute services

Medicare Part B: A supplemental program covering physician and other services and medical supplies

Medicare Part C: Medicare Advantage Insurance Plans

Medicare Part D: Supplemental coverage for drugs

MedPac: Medicare Payment Advisory Committee, a congressional agency

OCED: Off-campus emergency department

OPPS: Outpatient prospective payment system

PAC: Post-acute care provider

PCORI: Patient Centered Outcomes Research Institute

PFS: Physician fee schedule

PPACA: Patient Protection and Affordable Care Act (ACA for short)

PPS: Prospective payment system; rates set in advance rather than retrospectively based on costs

SNF: Skilled nursing facility

SSA: Social Security Act

UCC: Urgent care center

Notes

[1] Kate Davidson, "Social Security Costs to Exceed Income in 2020, Trustees Say," *Wall Street Journal* (April 22, 2019). The trustees add that the trust fund will be depleted by 2035.

[2] Anne Tergesen, "Medicare B Costs for Retirees Projected to Rise; Rising health-care prices at levels that 'exceed overall inflation' cited for increase," *Wall Street Journal* (April 22, 2019), https://www.wsj.com/articles/medicare-b-costs-for-retirees-projected-to-rise-11555978694?mod=searchresults&page=1&pos=1.

[3] Joseph Walker, "Why Americans Spend So Much on Health Care—In 12 Charts," *The Wall Street Journal* (July 31, 2018), https://www.wsj.com/articles/why-americans-spend-so-much-on-health-care-in-12-charts-1533047243.

[4] According to the MedPac website (www.medpac.gov), the Comptroller General of the United States is responsible for appointing individuals to serve as members of the Medicare Payment Advisory Commission (MedPac), an agency of Congress whose mandate is to analyze access to care, quality of care, and other issues affecting Medicare and to advise Congress on payments to health plans participating in the Medicare Advantage program and providers in Medicare's traditional fee-for-service program. MedPac was established by the Balanced Budget Act of 1997 (42 U.S.C. 1395b-6 (2008)). The commission's seventeen members serve three-year (renewable) terms (from May 1 to April 30). The law requires that the commission comprise a mix of individuals with expertise in the financing and delivery of healthcare services and have a broad geographic representation. Commissioners include physicians and other health professionals, employers, third-party payers, researchers with a variety of health-related expertise, and representatives of consumers and the elderly. In addition to the commissioners, there is a staff consisting of Executive and Deputy Directors, about 22 analysts and research associates, and about six other administrative staff. Although constituted as independent commission, the acknowledgments contained in the covering letter accompanying each MedPac report reveals the extent to which the Center for Medicare and Medicaid Services (CMS) staff provides "assistance." For instance, the 2010 MedPac report formally acknowledged assistance from 26 CMS staff and 50 others in government. Thus, it is subject to influence from these bureaucrats.

[5] MedPac, *Report to the Congress: Medicare Payment Policy* (March 2019), xiv, 8, 7, http://www.MedPac.gov/docs/default-source/reports/mar19_MedPac_entirereport_sec.pdf?sfvrsn=0.

[6] Jeff Desjardins, "The U.S. Spends More Public Money on Healthcare Than Sweden of Canada," *Visual Capitalist* (March 31, 2017), https://www.visualcapitalist.com/u-s-spends-public-money-health-care-sweden-canada/.

[7] Rachel Gillett, "The largest employers in each US state," *Business Insider* (June 11, 2017).

[8] "Here's a list of the largest employer in every state," *USA Today* (March 30, 2019).

[9] "The University's Economic Impact," *Rochester Review* (July-August 2018), 10-11, https://www.rochester.edu/pr/Review/pdfs/rr_july-august2018.pdf.

[10] Melanie Evans, "Midwest Hospital Systems to Merge Into 26-State Regional Giant," *Wall Street Journal* (June 28, 2019), https://www.wsj.com/articles/midwest-hospital-systems-to-merge-into-26-state-regional-giant-11561694580.

[11] MedPac (March 2019), 16, 17.

[12] Melanie Evans, "What Does Knee Surgery Cost? Few Know, and That's a Problem," *Wall Street Journal* (August 21, 2018), https://www.wsj.com/articles/what-does-knee-surgery-cost-few-know-and-thats-a-problem-1534865358.

[13] Evans (August 21, 2018), https://www.wsj.com/articles/what-does-knee-surgery-cost-few-know-and-thats-a-problem-1534865358.

[14] Anna Wilde Mathew, with contributions by Melanie Evans, "Secret Hospital Deals that Squelch Competition," *Wall Street Journal* (September 18 2018).

[15] Michael E. Porter and Elizabeth Olmsted Teisberg, *Refining Health Care: Creating Value-Based Competition on Results* (Cambridge, MA: Harvard Business Review Press, 2006).

[16] MedPac (March 2019), 11.

[17] MedPac (March 2019), 70.

[18] MedPac (March 2019), xiii.

[19] MedPac (March 2019), 9.

[20] Health Care Cost Institute 2016, MedPac, (March 2017), http://medpac.gov/docs/default-source/reports/mar17_entirereport.pdf.

[21] MedPac (March 2019), 16.

[22] Gretchen Jacobson, Meredith Freed, Anthony Damico, and Tricia Neuman, "A Dozen Facts About Medicare Advantage in 2019," Kaiser Family Foundation (June 6, 2019).

[23] MedPac (March 2001), 7 and 4; MedPac (June 2006), xvii; MedPac (March 2007), 16.

[24] National Conference of State Legislatures, "CON—Certificate of Need State Laws" (December 1, 2019), https://www.ncsl.org/research/health/con-certificate-of-need-state-laws.aspx.

[25] Neal Inman, "Certificat of Need: Doed It Actually Control Healthcare Costs?" Civitas Institute (September 14, 2011), https://www.nccivitas.org/2011/certificate-of-need-does-it-actually-control-healthcare-costs/.

[26] MedPac report (June 2006), xvii; MedPac report (March 2007), 16.

[27] MedPac report (March 2007), 16.

[28] Robert Ball, "What Medicare's Architects Had in Mind,"(*Health Affairs,* 14: 4 (1995), 67. 69; MedPac report (March 2007).

[29] MedPac report (2007), 5.

[30] Bob Rosenblatt, "Covered: A Week-by-Week Look at the 1965 Politics that Created Medicare and Medicaid," *National Academy of Social Insurance* (January 10, 2015), https://www.nasi.org/discuss/2015/01/covered-week-week-look-1965-politics-created-medicare-medica.

[31] Wilbur J. Cohen, "Reflections on the Enactment of Medicare and Medicaid," *Health Care Financing Review* (February 1, 1985), 5.

[32] Ball (1995), 69.

[33] Wilbur J. Cohen and Robert M. Ball, "Social Security Amendments of 1965: Summary and Legislative History," *Social Security Bulletin* (September 1965), 12, https://www.ssa.gov/policy/docs/ssb/

v28n9/v28n9p3.pdf.

[34] MedPac report (March 2007), 13.

[35] Cohen (February 1, 1985), 9.

[36] Stephen George Anastos, Jr., *Selling Medicare, Forgetting Medicaid 1960-1967,* Bachelor of Arts honors thesis, Harvard University (March 10, 2011), 102-120.

[37] Anastos quoting from Natalie Jaffe, "Medicare Revolution," *New York Times* (February 7, 1966), ProQuest Historical Papers *The New York Times* (1851-2007), .22.

[38] Anastos quoting from John Sibley, "Medical Care Furor," *New York Times* (May 21, 1966), Pro-Quest Historical Papers *The New York Times* (1923-Current file), 14.

[39] Anastos quoting from Glen Elsasser, "U.S. Picks Up Tab, Puts N.Y. Medicare Over," *Chicago Tribune* (May 29, 1966), ProQuest Historical Newspapers *Chicago Tribune* (1849-1987), 5.

[40] John Steele Gordon, "A Short History of American Medical Insurance," *Imprimis* (September 2018), 47: 9, https://imprimis.hillsdale.edu/short-history-american-medical-insurance/.

[41] Robert Helms, "The Origins of Medicare," *AEI* (March 1, 1999).

[42] Rick Mayes, "The origins, development, and passage of Medicare's revolutionary prospective payment system," *Journal of the History of Medicine and Allied Sciences* (January 2007), 62: 1, 21-55.

[43] Kimberly Amadeo, "The Rising Cost of Health Care by Year and Its Causes, See for yourself if Obamacare increased Healthcare Costs," TheBalance.com (November 14, 2018).

[44] Med Pac (March 2000), 5.

[45] Mayes (January 2007).

[46] Med Pac (March 2000), 5.

[47] Med Pac (March 2001), 90

[48] Med Pac (March 2000), 4-5

[49] Med Pac (March 2001), 90.

[50] Med Pac (March 2000), 5.

[51] Med Pac (March 2001), xvii, 4.

[52] See Centers for Medicare & Medicaid Services, "Skilled Nursing Facility PPS," https://www.cms.gov/Medicare/Medicare-Fee-for-Service-Payment/SNFPPS, and *Federal Register,* "Medicare Program; Prospective Payment System and Consolidated Billing for Skilled Nursing Facilities; Updates to the Quality Reporting Program and Value-Based Purchasing Program for Federal Fiscal Year 2020: A Rule by the Centers for Medicare & Medicaid Services on 08/07/2019, https://www.federalregister.gov/documents/2019/08/07/2019-16485/medicare-program-prospective-payment-system-and-consolidated-billing-for-skilled-nursing-facilities.

[53] Med Pac (March 2000), 6.

[54] Med Pac (March 2000), 6-7.

[55] Med Pac (March 2000), 7.

[56] MedPac (March 2002), 4.

[57] MedPac (March 2002), 3.

[58] MedPac (March 2018), 69.

[59] MedPac (March 2001), 5.

[60] MedPac (March 2001), 14-15.

[61] MedPac (March 2001), 16.

[62] MedPac (March 2001), 16.

[63] MedPac (March 2001), 89.,

[64] MedPac (March 2001), xix, 91.

[65] MedPac (March 2001), 186-187.

[66] MedPac (March 2001), 7.

[67] MedPac (March 2002), 5.

[68] MedPac (March 2001), 8; MedPac (March 2002), 5.

[69] MedPac (March 2002), xvi.

[70] MedPac (March 2002), 5; MedPac (March 2002), 43.

[71] MedPac (March 2002), 7; MedPac (March 2001), 5.

[72] MedPac (March 2007), xi, 9, 12.

[73] MedPac (March 2007), xiii.

[74] MedPac (March 2007), 22.

[75] MedPac (March 2007), 23.

[76] MedPac (March 2007), 21, 25.

[77] MedPac (March 2007), 25, 23.

[78] MedPac (March 2007), 25.

[79] MedPac (March 2007), xi, 5.

[80] MedPac (March 2007), xii, 47, xiii.

[81] MedPac (March 2007), xiii.

[82] MedPac (June 2008), xi, 7; MedPac (March 2009), 22.

[83] MedPac (March 2009), 58, 59.

[84] MedPac (March 2009), 57

[85] MedPac (March 2009), 5, 8.

[86] MedPac (March 2009), 9, 11.

[87] MedPac (March 2009), 12, 15, xiii, 39, 46, 47.

[88] "Evaluation of the Medicare Physician Group Practice Demonstration: Final Report" (September 2012), Prepared by RTI International, pp. ES-6 to ES-9.

[89] MedPac (March 2009), 47.

[90] MedPac (March 2006), 14; MedPac (March 2007), xiii; MedPac (March 2008), xii.

[91] MedPac (June 2008), 15, 87, 85, 83, 16, 83.

[92] MedPac (June 2008), 85, 87, 85.

[93] American Hospital Association, *Bundled Payment: AHA Research Synthesis Report,* https://www.aha.org/ahahret-guides/2010-03-01-bundled-payment-aha-research-synthesis-report, 4, 2, 5, 3, 12

[94] American Hospital Association, 9, 10.

[95] MedPac (June 2008), 87; American Hospital Association, 6.

[96] Glenn Hackbarth, covering letter, MedPac (March 2010).

[97] MedPac (June 2008), 16

[98] MedPac (June 2008), 73, 74, 66, 74.

[99] MedPac (June 2008), 173, 176, 175.

[100] MedPac MedPac (June 2008), 194, 176, 194, 195, 191-192.

[101] MedPac (March 2009), 22; Hackbarth, covering letter, MedPac (March 2010).

[102] Hackbarth, covering letter, MedPac (March 2010).

[103] John Cannan, "A Legislative History of the Affordable Care ACT: How Legislative Procedure Shapes Legislative History," *Law Library Journal* (July 2013), vol. 105, no. 2, 131-173.

[104] Glenn Kessler, "History Lesson: How the Democrats pushed Obamacare through the Senate," *Washington Post* (June 22, 2017), https://www.washingtonpost.com/news/fact-checker/wp/2017/06/22/history-lesson-how-the-democrats-pushed-obamacare-through-the-senate/.

[105] Cannan, op. cit.

[106] Cannan, op. cit.

[107] Cannan, op. cit.

[108] MedPac (March 2010), covering letter; MedPac (March 2007), 5.

[109] The official text of the ACA (Public Law 111-148—March 23, 2012) is found at https://www.govinfo.gov/content/pkg/PLAW-111publ148/pdf/PLAW-111publ148.pdf. The official text of the Reconciliation Act (Public Law 111-152—March 30, 2010) is at https://www.govinfo.gov/content/pkg/PLAW-111publ152/pdf/PLAW-111publ152.pdf.

[110] MedPac (March 2012), Executive Summary.

[111] General Accounting Office, "CMS Innovation Center: Model Implementation and Center Performance," GAO 18-302 (March 2018).

[112] MedPac (March 2005), 55.

[113] MedPac (March 2009), 15, 22, 12.

[114] The Physicians Foundation, "Health Reform and the Decline of Physician Private Practice: A White Paper Examining the Effects of the Patient Protection and Affordable Care Act on Physician Practices in the United States (Merritt Hawkins, 2010).

[115] NAACOS, website, www.naacos.com.

[116] Ibid.

[117] "What GAO Found" and p. 15 in General Accounting Office, "CMS Innovation Center: Model Implementation and Center Performance," GAO 18-302 (March 2018).

[118] General Accounting Office, "CMS Innovation Center: Model Implementation and Center Performance," GAO 18-302 (March 2018), 17-19.

[119] General Accounting Office, 32 and 33.

[120] MedPac (June 2018), 223, 211, 219.

[121] MedPac (June 2018), 230, 218.

[122] MedPac (June 2018), 230.

[123] Lewin Group, *CMS Bundled Payments for Care Improvement Initiative Models 2-4: Year 3 Evalua-*

tion & Monitoring Annual Report (October 2017—Revised October 2018).

[124] General Accounting Office, 34 and 35; Lewin Group, *CMS Bundled Payments for Care Improvement Initiative Models 2-4: Year 3 Evaluation & Monitoring Annual Report* (Final, October 2018), 265.

[125] U.S. Department of Health and Human Services, "Report to Congress: Evaluation of the Independence at Home Demonstration" (November 2018), 6, 9.

[126] General Accounting Office, 43.

[127] U.S. Department of Health and Human Services, Office of the Assistant Secretary for Planning and Evaluation, "Report to Congress on the Medicaid Health Home State Plan Option," as required by Section 2703 of the PPACA, and based on 5 annual reports done under contract by the Urban Institute (May 2018), 1, 2, 4.

[128] Ibid.

[129] MedPac (June 2018), 251-256.

[130] General Accounting Office, 36 and 43.

[131] General Accounting Office, 36 .

[132] General Accounting Office, 43

[133] General Accounting Office, 38

[134] General Accounting Office, 38, 39

[135] Melanie Evans, "What Does Knee Surgery Cost? Few Know, and That's a Problem," *Wall Street Journal* (August 21, 2018), https://www.wsj.com/articles/what-does-knee-surgery-cost-few-know-and-thats-a-problem-1534865358.

[136] General Accounting Office, "GAO Report to Congressional Committees. Comparative Effectiveness Research: Activities Funded by the Patient-Centered Outcomes Research Trust Fund," GAO-18-311 (March 2018), 12.

[137] General Accounting Office, (March 2018), 18.

[138] General Accounting Office, (March 2018), 8.

[139] MedPac (June 2018), 112.

[140] MedPac (June 2018), 118.

[141] MedPac (June 2018), 124.

[142] MedPac (June 2018), 179.

[143] MedPac (June 2018), 177.

[144] MedPac (June 2018), 177.

[145] MedPac (June 2018), 179.

[146] MedPac (June 2018), 112, 121.

[147] MedPac (June 2018), 123, 121, 133

[148] MedPac (March 2019), xiii.

[149] MedPac (March 2018), 69.

[150] MedPac (March 2019), 429.

[151] Medpac (June 2018), xvii.

[152] MedPac (March 2018), xviii, 183.

[153] MedPac (March 2018), xviii, xxiii.

[154] MedPac (March 2018), 191.

[155] MedPac (March 2018), 186, 188, 54, 184.

[156] MedPac (March 2018), 191.

[157] MedPac (March 2018), 191.

[158] MedPac (March 2018), 191.

[159] MedPac (March 2002), xv.

[160] MedPac (March 2019), 211, 203.

[161] MedPac (March 2019), 234, 231, 232.

[162] MedPac (March 2002), xvi; MedPac (March 2019), 228.

[163] MedPac (March 2018), 248.

[164] MedPac (March 2019), 242.

[165] MedPac (March 2019), 187.

[166] MedPac (March 2018), 277.

[167] MedPac (March 2019), 4, 61, 191, 61, 308.

[168] MedPac (March 2002), xiv.

[169] MedPac (March 2018), 118. The concern would be cited again on p. 117 of the March 2019 MedPac report.

[170] MedPac (March 2018), xxv, xxvi, 446.

[171] MedPac (March 2018), 129.

[172] MedPac (March 2009), 82.

[173] MedPac (March 2018), 129, 130.

[174] MedPac (March 2018), 129-130.

[175] MedPac (March 2018), 140.

[176] MedPac (March 2019), 140.

[177] MedPac (March 2019), 61.

[178] MedPac (March 2019), 61.

[179] Some politicians believe that government-regulated healthcare would be improved by simply allocating money to the states and leaving it up to them to run things. Even in this scenario, however, the federal government still sets the formulas for the states to obtain reimbursement for Medicaid expenditures, and the games the states can play to increase reimbursement have no end. CMS has a Federal Bonus Program called the Nursing Facility Upper Payment Limit. New York and other states set a fee (tax) on SNF private revenues because the intake of these funds leads to higher federal funding under the program. Other states like Indiana and Oklahoma have taken advantage of another opportunity to gain extra reimbursement for municipally owned nursing facilities.

On September 19, 2018, Paul Monies, a reporter for *Oklahoma Watch,* provided a prime example of how government-administered pricing leads to ridiculous consequences., whether that government is federal or state:

> He noted that a handful of small Oklahoma cities have become owners of dozens of nursing homes in the past couple of years simply to tap into a complex federal Medicaid reimbursement formula that should result in about 25% more revenue under this government ownership than under the previous

private ownership. As of the date of the article, the city of Pauls Valley owned licenses for 28 nursing homes that were scattered all over the state. The city of Hugo had nine licenses. Since the cities don't wish to actually operate the facilities, they typically sign management contracts with the previous owners, and negotiate what percentage of the increased rate each party is to receive. For their effort, the cities expect to receive millions more revenue. The scheme backfired in that CMS never approved the program, and as Barry Porterfield of the Pauls Valley Democrat wrote on June 15, 2019, the city transferred 13 of the 28 licenses back to the previous owners. However, the cities are still trying to get their scheme approved.

The state of Indiana provides another, and perhaps greatest example of this rate maneuvering. On Oct. 18, 2017 Phil Galewitz of Kaiser Health News reported that a drive to take advantage of the same quirk in the reimbursement formula has led to a situation in which nearly 90 percent of the state's 554 nursing homes have been leased or sold to county hospitals bringing in hundreds of millions in extra federal payments to the state. The state receives a marginal rate increase of approximately 30% over what the nursing homes previously received. If the facility is leased from the previous owners, the owner typically gets around 25% of the rate increase. An article in the Indianapolis Star on March 15, 2020 titled "Nursing home residents in Indiana suffer as country hospitals rake in millions," written by Tony Cook, Tim Evans, and Emily Hopkins, stated that Indiana received $679 million last year in extra Medicaid payments from the scheme. Investigations are finding that at least $1 billion, and possibly $3 billion of this extra funding got diverted to the municipal hospitals since 2003, and that the nursing homes have very low quality of care ratings. The scheme was concocted by Matthew Gutwein, the chief executive of the Marion County's public health system 20 years ago.

The Kaiser article stated that advocates say it has been a key factor in helping to keep Indiana's city and county hospitals economically vital at a time when many rural hospitals nationwide are facing serious financial difficulties. Gregg Malot, director of business development at Pulaski Memorial Hospital in northern Indiana stated that his hospital acquired 10 nursing homes, which has led to additional revenue of about $2 million a year, helping to finance the hospital's obstetrics care, the purchase of an MRI machine, and a centralized telemetry unit to monitor patients. Steve Long, CEO of Hancock Regional Hospital in Greenfield, Ind., said his hospital recently built two fitness centers in the county with help from its extra Medicaid dollars. "This would not be possible without the additional funding."

[180] Anna Wilde Mathews, "Behind Your Rising Health-Care Bills: Secret Hospital Deals That Squelch Competition," *Wall Street Journal* (September 18, 2018), https://www.wsj.com/articles/behind-your-rising-health-care-bills-secret-hospital-deals-that-squelch-competition-1537281963.

[181] MedPac (March 2013), 50.

[182] MedPac (March 2019), 16.

[183] Tim Mullaney, "Changing M&A Trends Make Home Health a Hotter Acquisition Target," *Home Health Care News* (January 31, 2018).

[184] Mathews (September 18, 2018), https://www.wsj.com/articles/behind-your-rising-health-care-bills-secret-hospital-deals-that-squelch-competition-1537281963.

[185] MedPac (March 2018), 14.

[186] MedPac (March 2018), 14, 15, 17.

[187] MedPac (March 2019), 81.

[188] Shelby Livingston, ""Reigniting the Physicians Arms Race, Insurers Are Buying Practices," *Modern Healthcare* (June 2, 2018), https://www.modernhealthcare.com/article/20180602/NEWS/180609985/reigniting-the-physicians-arms-race-insurers-are-buying-practices.

[189] MedPac (March 2019), 16.

[190] MedPac (March 2019), 209, 212; MedPac (March 2018), 212.

[191] MedPac (March 2019), 243.

[192] MedPac (March 2019), 74.

[193] MedPac (March 2019), 111, 112.

[194] MedPac (June 2013), xii.

[195] MedPac (March 2019), 75.

[196] MedPac (March 2019), 73.

[197] MedPac (March 2018), 13, 54.

[198] MedPac (March 2019), 76-77, 74-75.

[199] MedPac (March 2019), 74.

[200] MedPac (June 2019), 382.

[201] MedPac (June 2019), 384.

[202] MedPac (June 2019), 384, 386.

[203] MedPac (June 2019), 386.

[204] MedPac (June 2018), xiii, 42, 44, xiii, 39.

[205] MedPac (June 2018), 43.

[206] MedPac (March 2002), xvi

[207] MedPac (March 2018), 72.

[208] MedPac (March 2019), 74.

[209] MedPac (March 2018), 72, 128.

[210] MedPac (March 2018), 136-137.

[211] MedPac (March 2018), 60.

[212] MedPac (March 2019), xiv.

[213] MedPac (March 2019), 60-61.

[214] MedPac (March 2019), 16, 17.

[215] MedPac (March 2012), 18.

[216] MedPac (March 2019), 36, 37, 39.

[217] MedPac (March 2019), 4.

[218] Robert Helms, "The Origins of Medicare," *AEI* (March 1, 1999).

[219] Anna Wilde Mathews and Joseph Walker, "Health Effort by Amazon, Others Aims to Succeed Where Others Have Failed," *Wall Street Journal* (February 1, 2018).

[220] Jamie Reno, "Is Walmart's New Full-Service Clinic the Future of Community?" *Healthcare Healthline* (September 27, 2019), quoting Marcus Osborne, vice-president, Walmart Health and Wellness program.

[221] Anna Wilde Mathews, "Clinics Owned by Insurers Challenge Doctors, Hospitals," *Wall Street Journal* (February 24, 2020).

[222] MedPac (June 2018), 138.

[223] MedPac (June 2018), 134.

[224] MedPac (June 2018), xvi, 137, 165.

[225] MedPac (June 2018), 165.

[226] MedPac (March 2009), 102, 41, 39.

Made in the USA
Middletown, DE
06 November 2020